Self-Assessment Color Review

Ornamental Fishes and Aquatic Invertebrates

Second Edition

Self-Assessment Color Review

Ornamental Fishes and Aquatic Invertebrates

Second Edition

Gregory A. Lewbart
MS, VMD, DiplACZM
Professor of Aquatic Animal Medicine
North Carolina State University
College of Veterinary Medicine
Raleigh, NC, USA

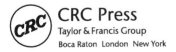

CRC Press
Taylor & Francis Group
Boca Raton London New York

CRC Press is an imprint of the
Taylor & Francis Group, an **informa** business

CRC Press
Taylor & Francis Group
6000 Broken Sound Parkway NW, Suite 300
Boca Raton, FL 33487-2742

© 2017 by Taylor & Francis Group, LLC
CRC Press is an imprint of Taylor & Francis Group, an Informa business

No claim to original U.S. Government works

Printed on acid-free paper
Version Date: 20160525

International Standard Book Number-13: 978-1-4822-5886-8 (Paperback)

This book contains information obtained from authentic and highly regarded sources. While all reasonable efforts have been made to publish reliable data and information, neither the author[s] nor the publisher can accept any legal responsibility or liability for any errors or omissions that may be made. The publishers wish to make clear that any views or opinions expressed in this book by individual editors, authors or contributors are personal to them and do not necessarily reflect the views/opinions of the publishers. The information or guidance contained in this book is intended for use by medical, scientific or health-care professionals and is provided strictly as a supplement to the medical or other professional's own judgement, their knowledge of the patient's medical history, relevant manufacturer's instructions and the appropriate best practice guidelines. Because of the rapid advances in medical science, any information or advice on dosages, procedures or diagnoses should be independently verified. The reader is strongly urged to consult the relevant national drug formulary and the drug companies' and device or material manufacturers' printed instructions, and their websites, before administering or utilizing any of the drugs, devices or materials mentioned in this book. This book does not indicate whether a particular treatment is appropriate or suitable for a particular individual. Ultimately it is the sole responsibility of the medical professional to make his or her own professional judgements, so as to advise and treat patients appropriately. The authors and publishers have also attempted to trace the copyright holders of all material reproduced in this publication and apologize to copyright holders if permission to publish in this form has not been obtained. If any copyright material has not been acknowledged please write and let us know so we may rectify in any future reprint.

Visit the Taylor & Francis Web site at
http://www.taylorandfrancis.com

and the CRC Press Web site at
http://www.crcpress.com

Dedication

To all of our patients: past, present, and future. They give so much and deserve our best.

Contents

Preface

There have been many exciting changes in ornamental fish and aquatic invertebrate medicine since I edited the 1998 version of this self-assessment guide. At that time there were far fewer veterinarians practicing fish medicine than there are today. Now virtually every major aquarium in the United States, and in many other countries, has at least one full time veterinarian, with some employing three or more. We have also witnessed an increased interest and awareness by traditional zoo veterinarians of the fish and invertebrate animals at their institutions. In addition to the International Association for Aquatic Animal Medicine (IAAAM), we now have the World Aquatic Veterinary Medical Association (WAVMA) and the American Association of Fish Veterinarians (AAFV). Veterinary participation in annual continuing education opportunities, such as the Eastern Fish Health Workshop, the Shark Reef Aquatic Medicine Seminar, and the Regional Aquatics Workshop (RAW), to list a few, is on the rise. These changes have allowed for an increased number of contributors to this edition while at the same time providing cases with more diagnostic and therapeutic depth and understanding.

Ornamental fish medicine is now included in many if not most veterinary curricula. This has sparked even more student interest in and awareness of fish and, in some cases, invertebrate medicine. There are also many more textbooks on these topics including at least two books on koi medicine alone. These factors combine to make the appearance of a second edition of this book both prudent and timely.

All of the cases and questions in this book are new, as are many of the contributors. Since this is a clinical work, the reader should keep in mind there can be more than one 'right' answer to many of the questions contained in these pages. In fact the reader may come across contradictory information and ideas when comparing similar case scenarios. This can be a healthy and constructive exercise and mimics what one sees in day-to-day veterinary practice.

I am indebted to the many knowledgeable contributors who so generously gave of their time. Without their breadth of knowledge and experience, this would not be the rich educational resource I hope the reader finds it to be.

Finally, as the editor of this work, I accept full responsibility for its content. Please use this book as a clinical guide, learning tool, and tank side resource. But do not rely on it as a stand-alone reference. Use your own clinical skills, intuition, and consultation with experienced colleagues before making real life clinical decisions on an unfamiliar case or medical challenge. And please take good notes and secure quality images when possible in order to help further advance fish and invertebrate medicine.

Good luck with all of your ornamental fish and aquatic invertebrate clinical efforts!

Gregory A. Lewbart

Contributors

Laura Adamovicz DVM
University of Illinois
Champagne, Illinois, USA

Lance Adams DVM
Aquarium of the Pacific
Long Beach, California, USA

Jeffrey R. Applegate Jr. DVM
North Carolina State University
College of Veterinary Medicine
Raleigh, North Carolina, USA

Shane Boylan DVM
South Carolina Aquarium
Charleston, South Carolina, USA

Terry W. Campbell MS, DVM, PhD
College of Veterinary Medicine
Colorado State University
Fort Collins, Colorado, USA

Julie M. Cavin DVM
New England Aquarium
Boston, Massachusetts, USA

Larry S. Christian BS
College of Veterinary Medicine
North Carolina Museum of Natural
Sciences
Raleigh, North Carolina, USA

Emily F. Christiansen DVM, MPH,
DiplACZM
North Carolina Aquariums
Raleigh, North Carolina, USA

Elsburgh O. Clarke III DVM
Audubon Aquarium of the Americas
New Orleans, Louisiana, USA

Tonya Clauss DVM, MS
Georgia Aquarium
Atlanta, Georgia, USA

Leigh Clayton DVM, DiplABVP
National Aquarium
Baltimore, Maryland, USA

Daniel S. Dombrowski MS, DVM
North Carolina Museum of
Natural Sciences
Raleigh, North Carolina, USA

Cara Field DVM, PhD
The Marine Mammal Center
Sausalito, California, USA

Robert H. George DVM
Ripley's Aquariums
Myrtle Beach, South Carolina, and
Gatlinburg, Tennessee, USA

Catherine Hadfield MA, VetMB,
MRCVS, DiplACVM, DiplECZM
National Aquarium
Baltimore, Maryland, USA

Craig A. Harms DVM, PhD, DiplACZM
College of Veterinary Medicine
Center for Marine Sciences and
Technology
North Carolina State University
Morehead City, North Carolina, USA

Tara M. Harrison DVM, MPVM,
DiplACZM, DiplACVPM
College of Veterinary Medicine
North Carolina State University
Raleigh, North Carolina, USA

Dan H. Johnson DVM, DiplABVP
Avian and Exotic Animal Care
Raleigh, North Carolina, USA

Rob Jones BVSc(Hons),
MACVSc(Aquatic Animal Health),
M. Aquaculture
"The Aquarium Vet"
Victoria, Australia

Lesanna L. Lahner DVM, MPH
Sealife Response, Rehabilitation,
  Research
Seattle, Washington, USA

Gregory A. Lewbart MS, VMD,
  DiplACZM
College of Veterinary Medicine
North Carolina State University
Raleigh, North Carolina, USA

Richmond Loh DipProjMgt,
  BSc, BVMS, MPhil(Pathology)
  Murdoch, MANZCVS(Aquatics
  & Pathobiology), CertAqV, NATA
  Signatory
The Fish Vet
Perth, Western Australia

Barbara Mangold DVM
Mount Pleasant Hospital for Animals
Newtown, Connecticut, USA

Stuart E. May BA
North Carolina Aquarium at Pine
  Knoll Shores
Pine Knoll Shores, North
  Carolina, USA

Alexa McDermott DVM
Georgia Aquarium
Atlanta, Georgia, USA

Blayk Michaels
Bass Pro Shops Base Camp
Springfield, Missouri, USA

Christine Molter BS, DVM
Houston Zoo, Inc.
Houston, Texas, USA

Brian Palmeiro DVM, DiplACVD
Pet Fish Doctor
Lehigh Valley Veterinary Dermatology
Allentown, Pennsylvania, USA

Ronald K. Passingham BS
College of Veterinary Medicine
North Carolina State University
Raleigh, North Carolina, USA

B. Denise Petty DVM
North Florida Aquatic Veterinary
  Services
Fort White, Florida, USA

Lysa Pam Posner DVM, DiplACVAA
College of Veterinary Medicine
North Carolina State University
Raleigh, North Carolina, USA

Komsin Sahatrakul DVM (Hons),
  CertAqV
Resorts World at Sentosa Pte. Ltd.
Singapore

Johnny Shelley MS, DVM, CertAqV
5-D Tropical Inc.
Plant City, Florida, USA

Donald Stremme VMD
AQUAVET®
College of Veterinary Medicine
Cornell University
Ithaca, New York, USA

Helen Sweeney DVM
Elma Animal Hospital
Aquatic Veterinary Services of WNY
West Seneca, New York, USA

William H. Wildgoose BVMS,
  CertFHP, MRCVS
Midland Veterinary Surgery
Leyton, London, UK

Roy P. E. Yanong VMD
Tropical Aquaculture Laboratory
Fisheries and Aquatic Sciences Program
School of Forest Resources and
  Conservation
IFAS/University of Florida
Ruskin, Florida, USA

Acknowledgments

I would first like to acknowledge the many individuals who have been a source of inspiration, support, and guidance. I thank all of my mentors and professors, but, in particular, Donald Abt, Robert Barnes, Philip Bookman, Dale Dickey, John Gratzek, Louis Leibovitz, William Medway, Trish Morse, Nathan "Doc" Riser, Ralph Sorensen, and Richard Wolke. I am fortunate to be associated with the North Carolina State University College of Veterinary Medicine (NCSU-CVM), a fine, progressive institution of higher learning. I am grateful to all of my NCSU-CVM friends and colleagues. Elizabeth Hardie, Craig Harms, Paul Lunn, Kent Passingham, and Michael Stoskopf have been especially supportive.

I collectively thank the veterinary students and house officers I have worked with, both at the NCSU-CVM and those from other colleges of veterinary medicine. These young people are the bright future of our profession, and on many days they teach me more than I teach them.

I am very grateful to the talented group of contributors who generously gave of their time and expertise to share their cases with you. I take full responsibility for any errors or omissions.

The folks at CRC Press have been exceptional through this entire process. I specifically acknowledge Jill Northcott, Commissioning Editor; Alice Oven, Senior Editor; Nikola Streak, who helped in the early stages; Julia Molloy, who was been patient, flexible, and responsive to queries; Helen Stanley and Peter Beynon, copy-editors extraordinaire; and Paul Bennett, Project Manager. I am fortunate and honored to have worked with Paul and Peter on both editions of this book.

Finally, I am grateful for the love, support, and wise insight provided by my wife, Diane Deresienski. She is always there to catch an idea or thought and toss back a strike, right down the middle.

Picture acknowledgments

The editor is grateful to the following for contributing figures to this book:

Alaska Sealife Center 73
S. Christian 194a, 194b
K. Hadfield 184b, 193
S. Hammer 206
C. Harms 159, 192b, 196a, 196b
K. Hartman 171a, 171b
L. Loh 184a
S. May 167
M. Mehalick 216a, 216b, 221

T. Miller-Morgan 182b
K. Passingham 217
D. Petty 5b, 139a, 139b, 154a–d, 170b, 175, 185, 191a, 191b, 192a
B. Phillips 177a, 177b, 220
F. Scharf 160a
J. Shelly 3
R. Vassallo 174c
L. Warren cover photo

Abbreviations

AST	aspartate aminotransferase	NSAID	non-steroidal anti-inflammatory drug
BAR	bright, alert, and responsive		
CBC	complete blood count	NSF	no significant findings
CK	creatine kinase	PCR	polymerase chain reaction
CNS	central nervous system	PCV	packed cell volume
CT	computed tomography	PO	per os, orally
DO	dissolved oxygen	ppm	parts per million
ERG	electroretinogram	ppt	parts per thousand
GA	general anesthesia	psi	pounds per square inch
GI	gastrointestinal	q	every
H&E	hematoxylin and eosin (stain)	sid	semel in die, 'once a day'
		TAN	total ammonia nitrogen
HLLE	head and lateral line erosion	TP	total protein
ICe	intracoelomic	TS	total solids
IM	intramuscular/intramuscularly	UV	ultraviolet
IV	intravenous/intravenously	WBC	white blood cell (count)

Broad classification of cases

Note: Some cases appear under more than one category.

Analgesia
37, 63, 67, 87, 147

Anatomy and physiology
1, 4, 6, 14, 19, 32, 39, 59, 64, 69, 73, 82, 86, 87, 89, 94, 97, 102, 106, 126, 136, 141, 162, 169, 177, 182, 189, 195, 197, 198, 199, 202, 214, 216, 221

Anesthesia
17, 30, 33, 34, 35, 43, 49, 50, 55, 60, 61, 62, 67, 69, 79, 88, 89, 104, 105, 111, 114, 136, 147, 197, 207, 213, 221

Bacterial diseases
12, 23, 46, 58, 62, 99, 108, 116, 119, 125, 152, 153, 163

Behavior
44, 51, 103

Buoyancy problems
51, 54, 92, 188

Cytology
5, 9, 10, 33, 49, 109, 148, 156, 159, 212

Environment/water quality
3, 7, 13, 15, 18, 39, 40, 41, 42, 44, 47, 52, 60, 71, 74, 76, 81, 83, 86, 88, 90, 91, 93, 96, 98, 99, 110, 115, 117, 118, 122, 131, 132, 133, 135, 136, 140, 141, 143, 145, 158, 161, 166, 167, 188, 196, 200, 206, 211, 217, 219

Filtration
9, 107, 165, 166, 179, 180, 183, 185, 190, 193, 203, 218

Fungal diseases
38, 56, 75, 104

Imaging
22, 29, 39, 45, 49, 54, 89, 94, 106, 135, 136, 141, 155, 157, 160, 169, 188, 198, 200

Neoplasia
21, 49, 79, 80, 105, 201

Nutrition
4, 5, 6, 14, 86, 110, 129, 149

Ophthalmology
8, 15, 18, 24, 25, 26, 146, 150

Parasitic diseases
1, 2, 11, 24, 25, 26, 27, 28, 30, 31, 53, 57, 65, 66, 70, 72, 77, 78, 84, 85, 92, 94, 100, 112, 113, 120, 121, 123, 127, 130, 137, 138, 142, 144, 150, 151, 154, 170, 171, 172, 173, 175, 176, 181, 184, 191, 192, 198, 204, 205, 210

Quarantine/transport
40, 41, 42, 215

Reproduction
22, 29, 59, 62

CASE 1 Six wild collected female bonnethead sharks (*Sphyrna tiburo*) have recently given birth in captivity. Animals were treated previously with 2.0 ppm praziquantel immersions of 7 days each and water quality shows no elevation in ammonia, nitrite, or nitrate. Three young bonnetheads have perished over the weekend and were observed eating during the week. The staff report nothing unusual on necropsy and the adults are eating and behaving normally. All sharks are swimming normally with no signs of dermatitis or ulceration. The tank temperature is 24.5°C (76°F). The staff are hesitant to capture the recently acquired adults.

1 What is your next diagnostic step considering the delicate nature of bonnethead sharks?
2 Had there been evidence of lactic acidosis, how would you manage this problem?

CASE 2
1 Why are there still monogeneans present in **Case 1** despite the praziquantel treatment and how will you proceed using the same drug?
2 What is the correlation between tank temperature and pathogen-induced dermatitis in the bonnethead sharks (*Sphyrna tiburo*) in **Case 1**?

CASE 3 A French grunt (*Haemulon flavolineatum*) weighing 2 kg is placed into an empty 1,500 L (395 US gal) hospital tank due to superficial traumatic abrasions and lacerations secondary to tank mate aggression. It is anesthetized, the lesions are treated, and empirical antibiotics and analgesics are started. The following morning the fish is found deceased on the bottom of the tank with flared gills.

1 What are your top differentials for the acute mortality?
2 What further testing do you want to do?
3 What abnormalities would you expect to find?
4 How would you manage the problem identified by your diagnostic work up?

CASE 4
1 How is the clinical presentation of goiter usually different in elasmobranchs as compared with bony fish?

1

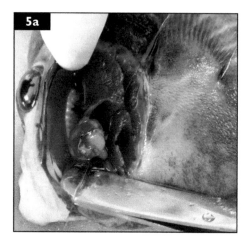

CASE 5 An angelfish (*Pterophyllum* sp.). from a large marine multispecies exhibit presents with a flared operculum. On sedation and examination it has a large fleshy mass originating from between the ventral gill arches (5a).

1 What is your top differential diagnosis?
2 What are your recommendations for treatment and prevention of this problem?

CASE 6 A 10-year-old blue ring angelfish (*Pomacanthus annularis*) presents freshly deceased for necropsy. Yesterday this fish was eating and acting normally

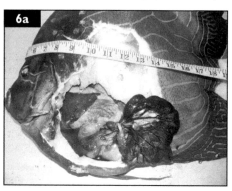

and the other fish in the system appear normal. There are no external problems identified and skin scrapes and gill clips are negative for parasitic disease. On opening the body cavity (6a) you find approximately 100 cc of blood tinged fluid and a foul odor.

1 Can you identify the pathologic lesion?

CASE 7 A lined seahorse (*Hippocampus erectus*) presents from the sygnathid exhibit in a public aquarium with multifocal 1–3 mm soft swellings of the skin along the snout. The seahorse was eating and behaving normally and had no lesions 24 hours ago.

1 What questions do you want to ask the aquarist?
2 What diagnostic tests do you want to perform?
3 Based on your findings what is the most likely diagnosis?

CASE 8 A bigeye *(Priacanthus arenatus)* presents with a diffusely cloudy cornea OD and distension of the globe. It has been eating well and behaving normally. It is housed in a mixed taxa exhibit with fiberglass habitat.

1 What diagnostics do you want to conduct?
2 What procedures and/or treatments would you perform?

CASE 9 A client presents a blue tang *(Paracanthurus hepatus)* for patches of skin that are losing color, particularly around the eye, and extending down the lateral line (**9a**). On examination the lesions are bilateral, slightly depressed, irregularly pigmented, and have smooth margins. There does not appear to be blood, increased mucus, or sloughing tissue associated with the lesions. You perform a skin scrape and find no metazoan parasites and cytology of the sample shows no bacteria and low cellularity.

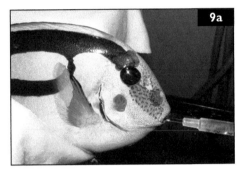

The owner tells you they have owned this fish for about 2 years but the lesions only began to develop over the last 2–3 weeks. The fish is housed in a 450 L (120 US gal) acrylic tank with a low density of other fish, no invertebrates, natural rock, and artificial coral pieces. Filtration equipment includes a canister filter, a wet dry trickle filter, and a UV sterilizer. The lighting is a fluorescent compact aquarium system and the bulbs were replaced within the last year. The water quality is tested weekly and is within appropriate levels, partial water changes are performed about every 14 days to keep the nitrate levels below 60 mg/L, and the tank is topped off with reverse osmosis water. The fish is fed a frozen and pelleted commercial diet for omnivorous marine fish and also eats a leaf of romaine lettuce a few times per week. When specifically asked about carbon filtration the owner tells you that he normally does not use carbon, but about a month ago the water in the tank was a bit yellow and carbon was added to the canister filter and in a net bag into the sump of the trickle filter. The water cleared up within 24 hours but the carbon is still in the filter.

1 What is the most likely diagnosis?
2 What questions would you like to ask the owner?
3 Describe HLLE for your client and provide information regarding prevention and treatment options.

CASE 10 A group of 30 pinfish (*Lagodon rhomboides*) were recently collected and brought into your collection. The animals were placed in an established quarantine system and routine quarantine treatment protocols were initiated. After 2 weeks you observe that multiple animals have developed multifocal white raised nodules along their dorsal, pectoral, and caudal fins (10). All animals are eating and swimming normally. There have been no mortalities noted.

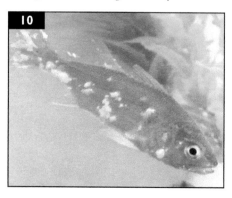

1 Is skin scraping these lesions appropriate?

You perform a skin scrape of the lesions and observe large fibroblasts on cytology. No ectoparasites are noted.

2 What is the top differential for these clinical signs and should the whole school of fish be culled and another batch obtained?

CASE 11 An aquarist brings you an Atlantic spadefish (*Chaetodipterus faber*), a marine fish, that had died earlier that morning. You perform a necropsy and on gill clippings you find multiple monogeneans presumed to be *Neobenedenia* sp. This animal is from a multispecies 756 L (200 US gal) marine exhibit displaying Atlantic blue crabs (*Callinectes sapidus*), spadefish, cobia (*Rhachycentron canadum*), and pinfish (*Lagodon rhomboides*). This exhibit shares the same filtration system with a large gallery that includes a touchpool exhibiting cownose rays (*Rhinoptera bonasus*), and several other exhibits that display speckled trout (*Cynoscion nebulosus*), red drum (*Sciaenops ocellatus*), sheepshead (*Archosargus probatocephalus*), and mullet (*Mugil cephalus*). The total amount of water in the system is 82,800 L (21,873 US gal).

1 Should the other exhibits in this system be suspected of having a monogenean infestation?
2 Would copper sulfate, a common drug used for treatment of ectoparasites, be indicated for use throughout the entire 82,800 L (21,875 US gal) system?
3 Devise a treatment plan for treating the entire system.
4 How much praziquantel would be needed for one treatment in the 82,800 L (21,875 US gal) system at a dosage of 2.5 mg/L?

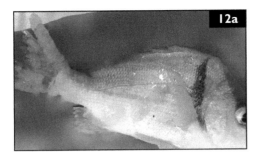

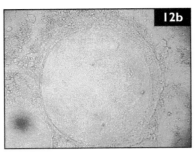

CASE 12 A population of 100 juvenile porkfish (*Anisotemus virginicus*) was introduced into a cownose ray (*Rhinoptera bonasus*) exhibit, but was removed 3 months later because the majority of these fish developed sores, growths, and frayed fins (**12a**). A wet mount image from a mucus smear made from one of the cutaneous lesions is shown (**12b**). The porkfish had nearly 100% morbidity with some fatalities, but the rays appeared healthy. During the following 10 days, the quarantined porkfish were treated with nitrofurazone (2–5 ppm as a prolonged immersion) for 5 days followed by formalin baths (250 ppm for 45 minutes) for 5 days and reduced salinity (15 ppt) with no response. During this period, there was 100% morbidity and the mortality rate was 30%. Treatment was switched to oxytetracycline (25 ppm as a prolonged immersion) and, after 5 days, there were only two mortalities and the remainder of the fish began to heal. During the following week the fish completely recovered and were returned to the exhibit.

1 Describe the lesions seen in **12a, b**.
2 What are the two most likely causes for the lesions seen in the porkfish?

CASE 13 An international shipment of marine tropical fish arrives after a 36-hour transit. On inspection the fish are normal in appearance and behavior. During the acclimation process the fish are placed in a bin with aeration and receiving tank water is slowly added to the shipping water. It is noted that some fish are lying on the bottom and all are respiring rapidly. A water sample initially collected from the shipping bag was analyzed for temperature 21.1°C (70°F), pH 5.8, oxygen saturation (92%), ammonia (>2.5 ppm), and nitrites (0.05 ppm).

1 Why are the fish developing these symptoms and what should be done to treat this problem and safely move forward with acclimation?
2 How could this problem be prevented with future shipments?

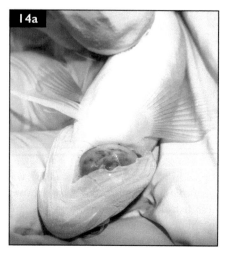

CASE 14 A yellowhead jawfish (*Opistognathus aurifrons*) presents with a flared right operculum. The fish completed routine quarantine without incident and has been housed in a 150 L (40 US gal) holding tank for the past month with one conspecific tankmate. A physical examination shows a 5 mm diameter light pink soft tissue mass medial to the right operculum and gills (**14a**). The appetite and chronicity of the mass is unknown as the fish is reclusive and often not seen for several days at a time. The fish appears to be in good body condition.

1 What are your top differentials?
2 What diagnostics do you want to perform?
3 Based on the results of your diagnostic tests what is the condition and how will you proceed?

CASE 15 An adult 12 g *Anthias* sp. from a mixed marine tropical fish tank presents with a severely enlarged right eye (**15a**). On closer examination you visualize a large amount of gas and trace amounts of blood within the eye. The remaining fish in the tank appear normal but there have been multiple previous cases of gas buphthalmia from this aquarium over the past year.

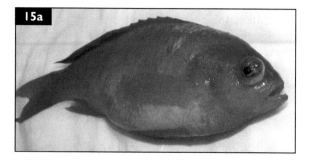

1 What are the possible causes for this condition?
2 What are the treatment options and prognosis for this fish?

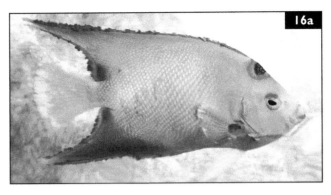

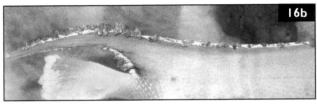

CASE 16 A cohort of five wild collected marine angelfish, including this queen angelfish (*Holacanthus ciliaris*) (**16a**), presented for medical evaluation following 2 weeks of isolation in a 1,100 L (290 US gal) quarantine system. All of these fish arrived at the facility in apparent good health. They were all maintained in the same quarantine system with adequate mechanical filtration. Over the course of approximately 1 week, three of the five fish developed wart-like masses (**16b**) within and circumscribing the outer edge of most fins, their mouths, and opercula. The fish were all eating well and were otherwise normal in behavior and attitude.

1 What diagnostic tests would you recommend?
2 Based on your findings what is your top differential diagnosis?
3 How would you manage this case?

CASE 17 Propofol has been used for anesthetizing fish.

1 What type of agent is propofol?
2 How can it be applied to fish?
3 Is this compound approved for use in fish intended for human consumption?

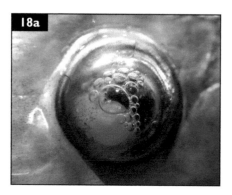

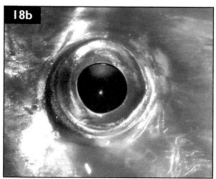

CASE 18 An adult lookdown (*Selene vomer*) maintained in a 35,000 L (9,245 US gal) mixed-species marine aquarium presented for medical evaluation of what was described as a 1-week history of gas bubbles observed in the right eye (**18a**). The left eye was reportedly normal (**18b**). The fish had been observed on multiple occasions over the past 2 weeks to be involved in extremely aggressive intraspecific interactions in the aquarium and was suspected to be reproductively mature. The aquarium was maintained with adequate mechanical and biological filtration. Other species in the aquarium included Florida pompano (*Trachinotus carolinus*), permit (*Trachinotus falcatus*), Atlantic spadefish (*Chaetodipterus faber*), red lionfish (*Pterois volitans*), and black sea bass (*Centropristis striata*). Other than the reported gas bubbles associated with the right eye, and increased fin damage linked to intraspecific tank-mate trauma, the fish was reported to be feeding and behaving normally. No new fish had been added to or removed from the system in several months. All other fish in the aquarium appeared healthy.

1 Describe the gross lesions present in **18a**.
2 What diagnostic tests would you like to employ other than physical examination?
3 Based on your diagnostic findings what is your diagnosis?
4 How will you manage the case?

CASE 19 You perform a necropsy on a recently deceased electric eel (*Electrophorus electricus*). During necropsy you cannot locate a cloacal opening (vent) along the ventrum of the animal.

1 Is this a pathologic or normal finding?

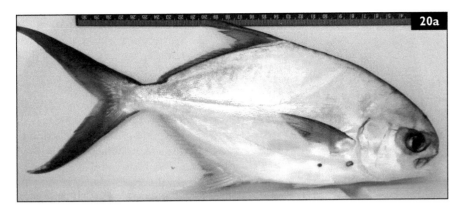

20a

CASE 20 An adult Florida pompano (*Trachinotus carolinus*) maintained in a 35,000 L (9,245 US gal) mixed-species marine aquarium presented for medical evaluation of what was described as a 1-week history of two small stable but non-healing ulcerative lesions located laterally below the right pectoral fin (20a). The aquarium was maintained with adequate mechanical and biological filtration. Other species in the aquarium included permit (*Trachinotus falcatus*), lookdown (*Selene vomer*), Atlantic spadefish (*Chaetodipterus faber*), red lionfish (*Pterois volitans*), and black sea bass (*Centropristis striata*). Other than the two described lesions, the fish were feeding and behaving normally over the past week. No new fish had been added to or removed from the system in several months.

1 To further evaluate this case, what approach would you take and what diagnostic tests would you recommend?
2 Based on your diagnostic findings how would you manage this case?
3 What aquarium inhabitant has most likely caused this injury?

CASE 21 An aquarist informs you that in the past month a large estuarine catfish (*Cnidoglanis macrocephalus*) that has lived in the aquarium for 5 years has an enlarged abdomen, a decreased appetite, and the fear is it is egg-bound. The other fish in the mixed display are fine and water quality parameters are normal.

1 How would you work this case up?
2 List your differential diagnoses.
3 What risks are involved with this species?

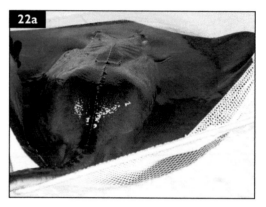

CASE 22 Aquarists request that you examine a 60 kg southern ray (*Dasyatis americana*) they think might be gravid (**22a**). The ray has had multiple litters of pups but due to exhibit overcrowding and the presence of male rays she was removed from the exhibit 2 years ago. When examined the ray is bilaterally swollen in the paralumbar areas as well as her abdomen.

1 What conditions would be on your rule out list and which is the most likely?
2 What diagnostic tests would you order?
3 If the ray is gravid, how would you explain that?
4 What other pathologic condition usually accompanies this clinical presentation?

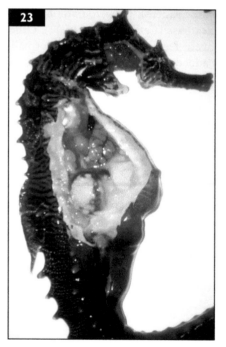

CASE 23 An aquarium facility has a large isolated 4,000 L (1,060 US gal) marine exhibit containing a large group of lined seahorses (*Hippocampus erectus*). An aquarist observes that an animal in the group has multiple erosive lesions along the dorsum and tail. The animal is euthanized. On necropsy you observe multiple large yellow granulomas within the coelomic cavity (**23**). You obtain an impression smear of the granulomatous lesions and apply an acid-fast stain. On 100× magnification you find acid-fast staining rods in various clumps.

1 What is the most likely diagnosis for this animal based on the impression smear?
2 What are some options that can be used to alleviate this diagnosis?

CASE 24 An emperor angelfish (*Pomacanthus imperator*) arrived in quarantine 1 month ago. Initial skin scrape, fin clip, and gill biopsy (s/f/g) revealed no parasites. The fish was treated with one round of praziquantel immersion as prophylaxis and was doing well in quarantine, but biologists noted the right pectoral fin and dorsal fin started to become tattered in appearance and the fish's right eye had become cloudy.

1 What are some differentials for the changes in the fish's appearance?
2 What diagnostics would you like to perform?

CASE 25 With regard to **Case 24**, after 2.5 minutes in a fresh water dip to treat ciliates, large white spots become evident on its eye and skin (**25a**). The white spots began to fall from the fish so you collect them from the bottom of the bucket and place them onto a slide. You find this parasite (**25b**).

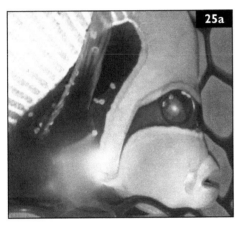 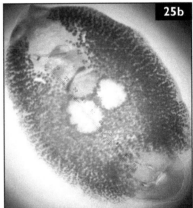

1 What parasite is this?
2 What treatment should be initiated?

CASE 26 The fish in **Case 25** is moved into a large multispecies exhibit. Three months after the fish was added you perform a necropsy on a fish that shares a tank with the angelfish. You find a severe *Neobenedenia* infection.

1 How did the parasite enter the system?
2 What is the next course of action?

CASE 27 An adult cownose ray (*Rhinoptera bonasus*) presents for weight loss and a wound on the pectoral girdle. Biologists report that the ray was recently introduced to the aquarium and is eating well. It is currently housed with 40 other cownose rays in a 14 m diameter round enclosure. On examination you notice that the dorsal surface of the ray is slightly pale, there are prominent lymphatic vessels, and the ray is very thin. On the ventral surface there is an ulcerative wound across the pectoral girdle. The ray appears active under manual restraint.

1 What questions would you like to ask the biologists?

CASE 28 With regard to **Case 27**, you learn the ray is swimming but appears to be lethargic and spends some time resting on the bottom of the enclosure.

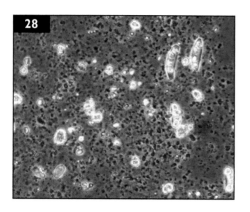

The rays are fed via broadcasting standard diet items into the enclosure. Biologists hand feed individuals that appear thin so they can ensure these animals are eating. The curators are reasonably certain this animal is eating well despite losing weight. The ray was recently wild caught in the Atlantic Ocean. A few other rays are demonstrating similar clinical signs. The water quality of the enclosure is acceptable.

1 What diagnostic tests would you recommend?
2 Microscopic evaluation of an aspirate reveals too numerous to count organisms of various life stages (**28**). What organism is this and what treatment should be initiated?

CASE 29 An ocean pout (*Zoarces americanus*) presents with a distended coelom of approximately 3 weeks' duration. It lives in a 9,500 L (2,500 US gal) mixed-species exhibit with sand bottom and minimal habitat. It is the only one of its species and has been eating well and behaving normally.

1 What are your top differentials?
2 What diagnostics do you want to pursue?
3 Once you have your diagnosis what are your treatment/management options?

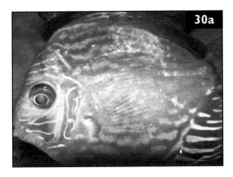

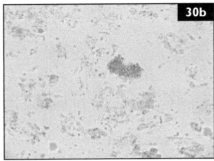

CASE 30 A discus (*Symphysodon aequifasciatus*) was brought to the hospital due to weight loss and scale erosion on the sides of the body, just dorsal to the lateral line (**30a**).

1 What are the top differentials for weight loss and scale erosion?
2 What type of diagnostics would you like to perform?
3 You place a fecal sample on a slide and note numerous swimming parasites (**30b**). What is the parasite seen on the slide?
4 How will you treat the fish?

CASE 31 A small group of lined seahorses (*Hippocampus erectus*) were obtained from a breeder and were mixed with another group of seahorses going through quarantine. One seahorse had a single white spot noted on the skin. Two weeks later that seahorse had multiple raised yellow-white spots in the skin, singly and in clusters (**31a**).

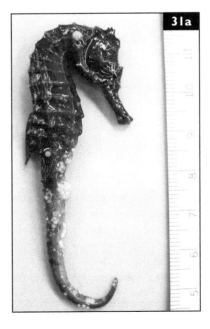

1 What is your presumptive diagnosis?
2 How do you confirm your presumptive diagnosis?
3 How will you manage the individual and the population?

13

CASE 32 A squirrelfish (*Holocentrus ascensionis*) presented to you for coelomic distension. Aquarists report that it has been this way for over 1 month but they were only now able to catch it for examination. You examine the fish and note that it is BAR, swimming normally, and respiring well. The eyes are clear bilaterally and there is no scale loss; you note that the coelom is severely distended.

1 What questions do you have for the aquarist?

CASE 33 The aquarist in **Case 32** reports that the fish is eating well and is of unknown sex. Other fish in the tank are exhibiting no abnormal clinical signs and the water quality is within normal limits. You decide the fish needs to have further diagnostics performed and the fish will need to be sedated. You are familiar with MS-222 so you sedate the fish with 60 ppm MS-222 buffered with bicarbonate. After a few minutes the fish is still swimming normally and will not allow you to handle it, therefore you add another 10 ppm MS-222 to the anesthesia tank. The fish begins to lose its equilibrium and lists to one side. Respiration remains spontaneous and regular.

1 What stage of anesthesia is the fish exhibiting?
2 How will you monitor anesthesia?
3 What diagnostics can you perform while the fish is under anesthesia?
4 What are your primary differentials for the coelomic distension?

CASE 34 With regard to **Case 33,** as there was no definitive diagnosis, you decide to perform an exploratory surgery to view the organs and possibly take biopsies.

1 What is your anesthetic plan?

CASE 35 The fish in **Case 34** was placed into the anesthetic water and 8 minutes later was sufficiently anesthetized for surgery. The fish was placed onto the surgical table in dorsal recumbency. No spontaneous gill ventilation was noted.

1 What do you do?
2 How do you prepare the fish for surgery?

CASE 36 Regarding the fish in **Case 35,** you open the coelomic cavity by making a stab incision (with a #15 blade) and extend the incision cranially and caudally using Metzenbaum scissors. You note the following on exploration: the stomach is distended and appears to contain food material; the intestines are also full of digesta. The coelomic wall is very thin and the surface has evidence of inflammation. The swim bladder, liver, and spleen all appear within normal limits. The ovaries are noted to be irregular in size and have ova present in various stages of development. Some follicles appear necrotic and are filled with yellow liquid.

1 What, if any, samples would you like to take?

CASE 37 Due to concern over possible contamination during surgery and from diseased ovarian tissue remnants, the fish in **Case 36** is started on antibiotics (20 mg/kg enrofloxacin diluted with sterile saline intracoelomically). The fish also received 0.1 mg/kg meloxicam IM for analgesia. Following surgery the fish is returned to a recovery bin with fresh saltwater. Her heart rate is strong and regular but she is not respiring on her own.

1 What do you do?
2 Given the discovery of abnormal ovaries, risk of infection, and high WBC count, what kind of post-surgical treatment is warranted?

CASE 38 An adult lumpfish or lumpsucker (*Cyclopterus lumpus*) in a cold marine exhibit is found dead in its exhibit. The two remaining fish are eating well and behaving normally, but are showing crateriform skin ulcers. The system has been stable and water quality parameters have been within normal limits. On necropsy, granuloma-like lesions and multifocal to coalescing black foci are seen in the viscera. Fungal hyphae are found on impression smears of the skin lesions and viscera (**38**).

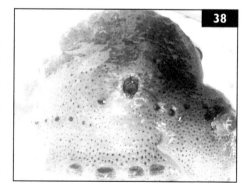

1 Cultures and sequencing are pending, but what is the likely diagnosis?
2 What is the prognosis?

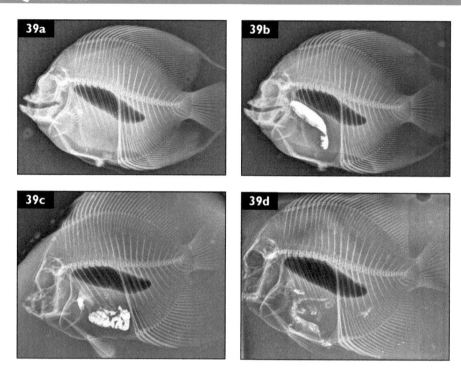

CASE 39 A French angelfish (*Pomacanthus paru*) arrived from another facility in apparently good health and started eating the following day. One week later it stopped eating and the aquarist reported it was occasionally twitching. Examination, including skin scrape, gill clip, and fin clip as well as visual physical examination, revealed no abnormalities, and the fish was in good body condition with normal coloration. The next day the aquarist reported that the cloaca looked distended with exposed tissue. The fish was anesthetized and the cloaca was noted to be mildly swollen, but not prolapsed, and a thin strand of foreign material similar to fishing line was present within the vent.

1 List some of the details about this animal's history you would like to know?
2 What should you do next?
3 Are there any abnormalities on this radiograph (**39a**)?
4 Does this fish have an obstruction (**39b–d**)?

CASE 40 A shipment of tetras was supposed to arrive at your facility today (a hot summer day) but you learn the shipment is delayed 24 hours.

1 What are your concerns for the fish?

CASE 41 On arrival at your facility you note that approximately 30% of the fish in **Case 40** are dead. The deceased fish are severely autolyzed so you are unable to perform a productive necropsy. Water quality of the shipment water is examined, and the ammonia is high, the water temperature is elevated, and the DO is low.

1 What, if anything, can you do to help the remaining fish survive?

CASE 42 Unfortunately, fish in **Case 41** keep dying at a high rate. You decide to euthanize some moribund fish for necropsy. Skin scrape, fin clip, and gill biopsy reveal no pathogens. Histopathology results come back and suggest a water-borne irritant that caused severe gill damage.

1 What is your next treatment plan?

CASE 43 A 2.85 kg freshwater drum (*Aplodinotus grunniens*) living in a large public exhibit presented for a raised, pale, dorsal periorbital swelling of the left eye (**43a**).

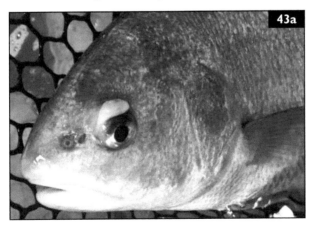

1 What would be your diagnostic plan?
2 How would you manage this case?

CASE 44 You work at a facility that houses several different species of seahorses. Water quality parameters are stable and the population appears healthy in general. One day an aquarist informs you that one of the adult male seahorses is floating on its side at the surface; when she touched it to see if it was alive it was still able to swim around. The other seahorses sharing its enclosure are fine.

1 What steps should you take to work up this case? What diagnostic procedures would you like to perform?

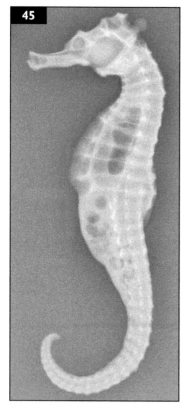

CASE 45 On visual assessment the animal in Case 44 is upright and grasping a piece of décor with its tail. It does not have any skin lesions or other obvious physical abnormalities, although it seems to be respiring more quickly than the others. You gently release it from the décor and it swims away initially but then floats to the surface where it stops actively swimming. You bring the seahorse to your examination room for radiography (45).

1 Describe your findings.
2 What are some possible reasons for this condition and what treatments can you apply?

CASE 46 When dealing with the same system as in Case 45, the next week the seahorse aquarist reports that one of the females in a different system is lying on her side on the bottom of the exhibit and has not eaten in several days. You perform the same examination and diagnostic procedures as with your last seahorse patient and find a small ulcerated lesion on the side of the fish, observe an increased respiratory rate, and a seahorse reluctant to move. You collect a skin scrape of the lesion and see blood cells, mucus, and large numbers of mixed bacteria. Slides are prepared for staining and you obtain radiographs of the seahorse.

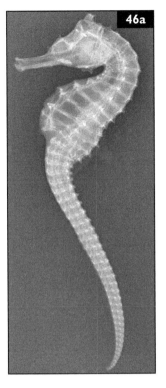

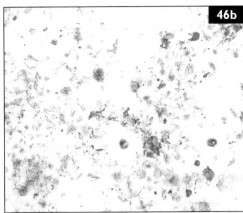

1 Describe the radiographic findings (46a).
2 What three basic stains can you use to help evaluate the skin lesion?
3 The acid-fast stained slide is shown (46b). What is your top differential based on this result?

CASE 47 A large saltwater fish system is showing acute mortalities involving the pelagic fish. Other fish in the system are lethargic and low in the water column. Microbubbles are visible on the décor. At necropsy, the fish are in good condition, with digesta in the GI tract. Lesions are seen on the gills (47) and fins.

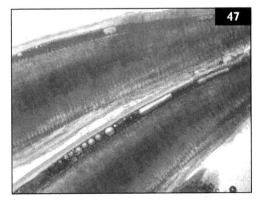

1 What is the likely problem?
2 What tests could confirm your diagnosis?
3 List possible etiologies.

CASE 48 A sub-adult lesser amberjack (*Seriola fasciata*) presented with a mass on the left operculum, just caudal to the commissure of the mouth,

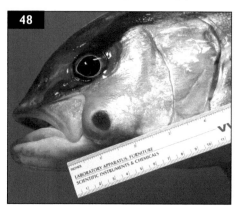

approximately 3.5 cm ventral to the eye (48). The fish was in good body condition, behaved normally, and appeared to have no issue prehending and ingesting food. No evidence of trauma or aggression had been noted. The mass enlarged progressively and the skin over the mass ulcerated.

1 What are some differentials for the cause of the mass and ulceration?

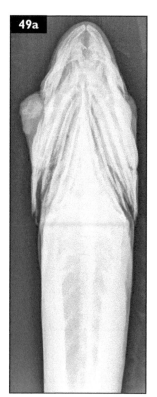

CASE 49 The fish in Case 48 was anesthetized with buffered MS-222 at 90 mg/L for examination and diagnostics. Radiographs (49a) revealed a discrete bone density mass.

1 In addition to radiographs, what other diagnostics or procedures could be performed while this fish is under anesthesia?

CASE 50 Eugenol (clove oil) has been used for anesthetizing fish.

1 What type of agent is eugenol?
2 How can it be applied to fish?
3 Is this compound approved for use in fish intended for human consumption?

CASE 51 In an established 220 L (58 US gal) tank with three oscars (*Astronotus ocellatus*) one fish presents with a loss of buoyancy control when at rest (**51**). The other two fish show no clinical signs.

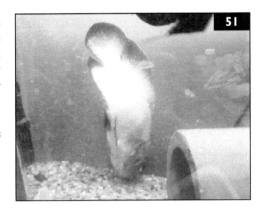

1 What are some potential causes for this problem?

CASE 52 In Case 51, it was found that nitrite levels were markedly elevated. After quizzing the owner, you realize she had changed to a new filter and had inadvertently created 'new tank syndrome' in an established aquarium.

1 What management and treatment options will you prescribe for nitrite toxicosis?
2 How might the owner avoid this situation in future?

CASE 53 Your facility is opening a jellyfish exhibit and a group of blubber jellies (*Catostylus mosaicus*) arrives in terrible shape. Physical examination reveals creatures within the bell of many individuals (**53**).

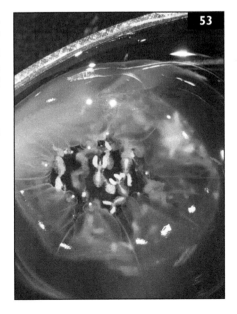

1 What are they and how would you treat them?

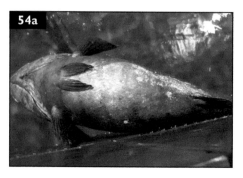

CASE 54 An 81 kg giant grouper (*Epinephelus lanceolatus*) was noted to be abnormally buoyant with difficulty maintaining an upright posture (**54a**). The coelom was markedly distended. Numerous bite wounds of varying severity were noted on the caudal peduncle. The fish was fairly unreactive when handled.

1 Describe an appropriate course of action to diagnose the problem(s).

CASE 55 Multiple pockets of free air were noted in the coelom of the fish in Case 54, with halo artifacts on ultrasound. The fish remained abnormally buoyant over the next 3 days despite three coelomic aspirations, each evacuating 200–300 ml of air. While anesthetized with 60 mg/L buffered MS-222, radiographs were obtained. The entire coelom appeared to be air filled.

1 What are some differentials for the cause of free air in the coelom of this fish?

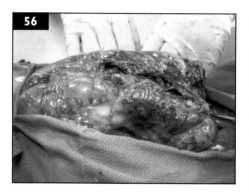

CASE 56 With no improvement by day 3, the fish in **Case 55** was anesthetized again. After aseptic surgical preparation an exploratory laparotomy was carried out. On entering the coelom, it was difficult to visualize organs (**56**), and abundant dark, discolored, foul smelling tissue protruded from the coelom with little manipulation. Due to poor prognosis, the fish was euthanized. Histopathology revealed granulomas within the swim bladder, spleen, and GI tract. Gomori-Grocott methenamine silver (GMS) and periodic acid–Schiff (PAS) stains revealed large numbers of septate hyphae with thin, non-parallel, 2–5 µm walls. Septation was common with segments of variable length and frequent bulbous swellings. Branching was infrequent.

1 What is the most likely cause of the disease process in this fish?

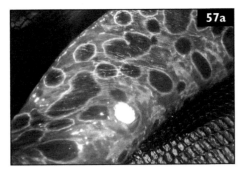

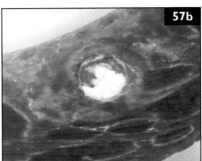

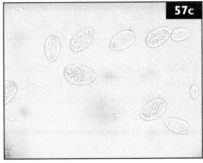

CASE 57 An aquarist tells you that a peacock wolf eel (*Anarrhichthys ocellatus*) has a discolored spot on the skin of its tail. The lesion is round, 1.5 cm wide, and very superficial with loss of just the epidermal layer (**57a**). You perform a skin scrape of the lesion and see only mucus and a few red and white blood cells. As the lesion is small and superficial, you decide to recheck it in a few days. When you recheck the wound 5 days later the wound is now 2 cm in diameter and extends into the deeper muscle tissue (**57b**). You perform another skin scrape (**57c**).

1 What are these organisms and why didn't you see them before?
2 What types of treatments are effective against this organism?

CASE 58 Koi (*Cyprinus carpio*) with aeromonad septicemia are being treated with antibiotics. Based on the antibiotic sensitivity panel, florfenicol was used to treat the fish by intramuscular injection at a dose of 30 mg/kg. All fish reacted adversely to the drug (**58**).

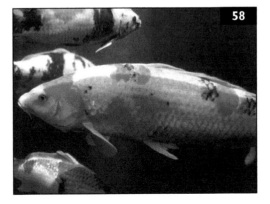

1 Describe the changes.
2 How would you remedy the situation?

23

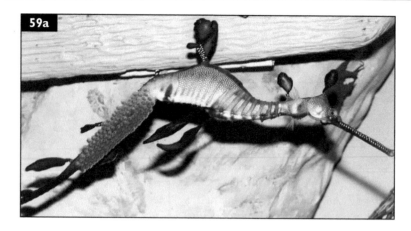

CASE 59 The owner of a public aquarium rings up and mentions that a weedy sea dragon (*Phyllopteryx taeniolatus*) has developed red bubbles on its tail overnight. The sea dragons have been in a monospecies tank that has been established for 5 years and the main issue has been some occasional scutociliate (protozoan) infections. You examine the fish (**59a**).

1 Is there a problem?

CASE 60 A 2.1 kg rainbow trout (*Oncorhynchus mykiss*) is displaying a pronounced triangular ventral distension just caudle to the pectoral fins (**60a**).

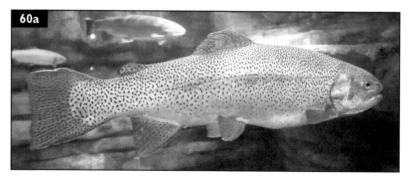

1 What would be the most pertinent questions to ask?
2 What examination technique would you recommend?

CASE 61

1 How would you manage the remaining affected trout from **Case 60**?

CASE 62 You are asked to assess a 15-year-old female sand tiger shark (*Carcharias taurus*) that has been on display for 6 years. She has been eating erratically for some time, is now anorexic, and recently developed dermal lesions (**62a**). All other sharks in the exhibit are normal. Water quality parameters are within normal limits. When restrained for a physical examination the animal is sedated with oxygen narcosis and tonic immobility. In addition to the dermal lesions you notice the shark's cloacal region is inflamed and the cloacal pores are enlarged and hyperemic (**62b**).

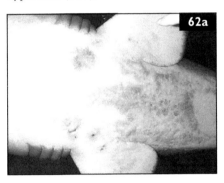 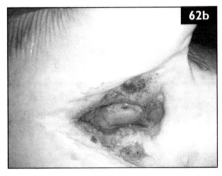

1 What are the skin lesions and what are their significance?
2 What would be your rule out list?
3 What diagnostic tests would you order?
4 How would you treat this case?

CASE 63 You have been asked to consult on a colleague's koi (*Cyprinus carpio*) abdominal surgery case that will be quite involved. Your colleague would like your input on developing an analgesic protocol.

1 What agents would you consider?
2 What are the advantages and disadvantages of each?
3 The client is looking for ways to minimize cost and asks your colleague if pain medications are needed; he has read that fish do not feel pain. How would you address this topic?

25

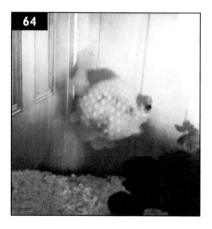

CASE 64 An adult goldfish (*Carassius auratus*) presents with multiple fluid-filled growths along its ventrum (**64**).

1 What breed of goldfish is this?
2 Identify the growths.

CASE 65 The owner of a 3,000 L (790 US gal) coral system has noticed little red spots on her *Acropora* spp. corals. The owner thinks the corals may be showing reduced polyp emergence and growth rates. Water quality has been within normal limits and the life support system is working adequately. The last animals added to the system were a mixture of hard corals about 2 months previously. A coral head was examined under the dissecting microscope (**65a**) and one of the parasites seen was examined under a higher-power microscope (**65b**).

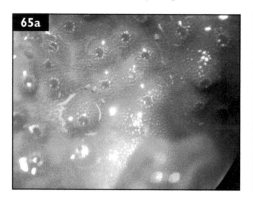
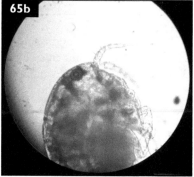

1 What is this parasite?
2 What is the host range?
3 What is the most common treatment used to control this parasite?

CASE 66 Several doctorfish (*Acanthurus chirurgus*) in a 7,000 L (1,850 US gal) saltwater quarantine system are lethargic, dark, and inappetent. The fish came from a commercial supplier 4 weeks previously and since arrival have been prophylactically treated with copper sulfate (0.18–0.20 mg/L immersion for 21 days). Water quality and temperature have been within normal limits. The life support system is working normally. On visual examination of the fish, clinical signs also include tachypnea, dyspnea, brown foci on the skin, and bilateral keratitis. On skin scrapes, increased mucus and rare parasites up to 3 mm in length are found (**66a**). On gill biopsies, triangular structures are seen ~120 μm in diameter (**66b**).

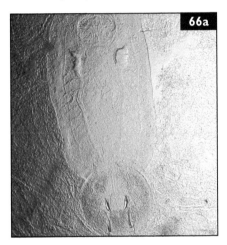 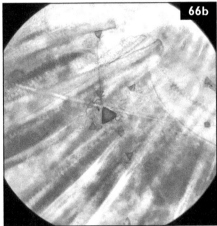

1 What is this parasite?
2 What is the significance of this parasite?
3 What treatment options would you consider?

CASE 67 Tricaine methanesulfonate (MS-222) is a commonly used fish anesthetic agent.

1 What type of agent is MS-222?
2 Is this compound acidic or basic and how would you bring a stock solution close to neutral?
3 What handling precautions should be taken and is this compound dangerous to humans?
4 Does MS-222 have analgesic properties?

CASE 68 A new jellyfish gallery is opening and specimens are arriving. A few days after a group of spotted jellies (*Mastigias papua*) arrives you note circular lesions on the bell that look as if the bell is melting.

1 How would you diagnose the problem and what are some possible etiologies?

CASE 69 The Port Jackson shark (*Heterodontus portusjacksoni*) is a member of the horn shark family (Heterodontidae) (**69a**). They are common in shallow, southern Australian waters, often resting on the bottom, and are commonly displayed in public aquaria. A juvenile was presented for a suspected GI prolapse. On examination a mass was present near the vent (**69b**, arrow).

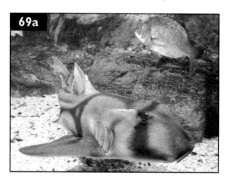

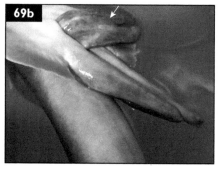

1 What would you do to examine further and make a diagnosis?
2 How would you resolve the problem?
3 What sex is this shark?

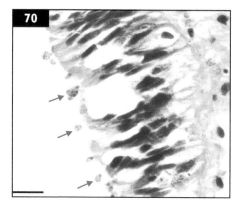

CASE 70 This parasite is often found on the gills of the giant Pacific octopus (*Enteroctopus dofleini*) (**70**, arrows). It is a commonly reported pathogen in teleosts.

1 What is it?

CASE 71 You are called to examine a 4,500 L (1,190 US gal) pond with 12 adult koi (*Cyprinus carpio*). The presenting complaint is mortality (50%), respiratory distress, lethargy, and abnormally appearing skin and fins (**71**).

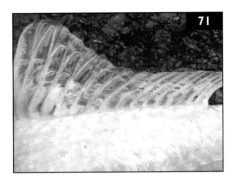

1 Describe the physical examination findings present.
2 What is your diagnosis?
3 Name potential causes for this condition.
4 How would you manage this problem?

CASE 72 Spotted seatrout (*Cynoscion nebulosus*), or speckled trout, collected for lab-based validation of a subsequent field telemetry project, develop blotchy skin and lethargy with some mortalities during an acclimation period. A moribund fish is euthanized for examination. You find necrosis of gill lamellae tips (**72a**) and perform microscopic examination of gill and skin scrape wet mounts (**72b**).

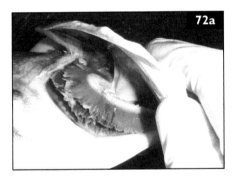 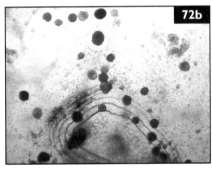

1 To what family do spotted seatrout belong?
2 What is the infesting organism and what are treatment options?

CASE 73 The giant Pacific octopus (*Enteroctopus dofleini*) is a popular exhibit animal in public display aquaria.

1 How can the sex of a giant Pacific octopus be determined?

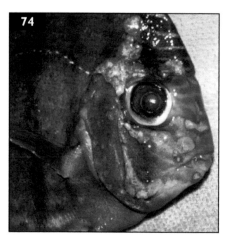

CASE 74 An adult discus (*Symphysodon* sp.) presents for symmetrical, depigmented coalescing erosions and ulcers producing crateriform lesions and pits on the head (**74**). There were five other discus in the population housed in a 415 L (110 US gal) aquarium. No other fish were affected.

1 What is the common name of this condition?
2 List possible underlying causes.
3 What are possible treatment options?

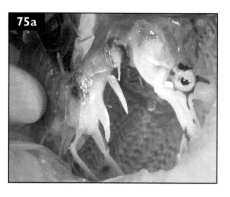

CASE 75 A leafy sea dragon (*Phycodurus eques*) is presented showing lethargy and anorexia for a few weeks. Two large black areas of eroded skin had appeared in the past few days (**75a**).

1 What diagnostic tests would you undertake to make a diagnosis?
2 What is the most likely diagnosis?
3 How do you treat this?

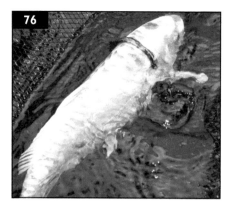

CASE 76 A single koi (*Cyprinus carpio*) presented suddenly with a green rubbery flap behind its head (**76**). The fish was otherwise behaving normally.

1 What could this be?

CASE 77 A quarantine tank of mixed marine species, including black drum (*Pogonius cromis*), permit (*Trachinotus falcatus*), Florida pompano (*Trachinotus carolinus*), harvestfish (*Peprilus alepidotus*), and lookdowns (*Selene vomer*), experience some epithelial hyperplasia and a high mortality rate. On a wet mount microscopic examination of skin scrapings from surviving fish you observe numerous flat ovoid to elongated organisms with two eyespots (**77a**). You subsequently observe low numbers of similar organisms (**77b** shows detail of the anterior end, with two eyespots and cilia visible along the margins of the organisms, 100×) during quarantine examinations of apparently healthy northern pipefish (*Syngnathus fuscus*, marine) and a long-term exhibit of white catfish (*Ictalurus catus*, freshwater; **77c**, 100×) with multicentric cutaneous lymphoma.

1 What is the organism?
2 How do you treat it?

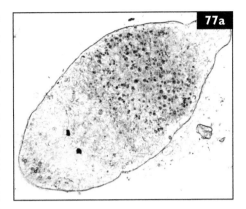

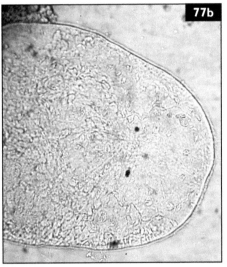

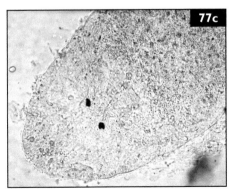

CASE 78 A concrete-lined pond with koi (*Cyprinus carpio*) was being treated for *Argulus* sp. (**78a, b**) using trichlorfon at a rate of 1.0 mg/L. However, it proved to be ineffective despite several doses.

1 Why might that be?
2 How would you manage the situation?

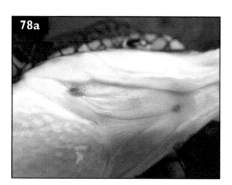
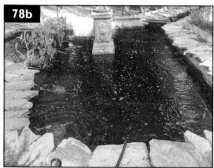

CASE 79 An adult koi (*Cyprinus carpio*) weighing 4.6 kg presented for an approximately 6-month history of a large pigmented mass dorsal to the right eye and caudal to the nare. The fish lived in a pond with other koi at a zoological institution. Appetite, activity level, and behavior were normal. The koi was anesthetized

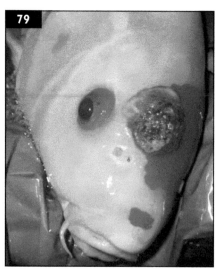

with sodium bicarbonate buffered tricaine methanesulfonate (MS-222) at 75 ppm. On physical examination the integumentary mass measured 2.5 cm in diameter, was raised, multipigmented, and friable (**79**). A CBC, biochemistry profile, gill clip cytology, skin scrape cytology, fecal parasite screen, and coelomic ultrasound were unremarkable. Radiographs indicated soft tissue swelling in the region of the mass, but no boney involvement.

1 What are your primary differentials for this lesion?
2 What is your diagnostic plan for this fish?

CASE 80 While under anesthesia the koi in **Case 79** had an excisional surgical biopsy. The tissue surrounding the mass was injected with 5 mg lidocaine hydrochloride and the skin was rinsed with sterile saline. The center of the mass was excised with a 3-0 polydioxanone (PDS II) suture using a guillotine-type method, leaving tissues at the margins circumferentially. The margins were cryoablated using liquid nitrogen with three blanche cycles. Healthy bone was exposed beneath the mass and was covered with 1% silver sulfadiazine cream. Ceftazidime and ketoprofen were also administered. The fish recovered without incident and was returned to its pond exhibit. The mass was submitted for histopathology and found to be a spindle cell neoplasm. This photomicrograph (**80a**, 40×) of the mass shows streams of neoplastic spindle cells with occasional pleomorphic multinucleated cells. Several spindle cell neoplasms are similar histologically and, for this case, may include a peripheral nerve sheath tumor, chromatophoroma (erythrophoroma, melanoma, or xanthophoroma), or mesenchymal tumor (fibrosarcoma). Further

testing, such as electron microscopy or immunohistochemistry, would be needed for a definitive diagnosis. Six months after initial presentation, the koi was clinically well, but had a ridge of proliferative tissue along the caudal edge of the former mass site (**80b**). The area of previously exposed bone was completely epithelialized. A portion of the proliferative tissue was surgically biopsied and submitted for histopathology. The remainder was cryoablated using liquid nitrogen with three blanche cycles. Histopathology indicated recurrence of a spindle cell neoplasm.

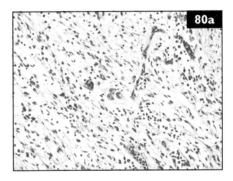

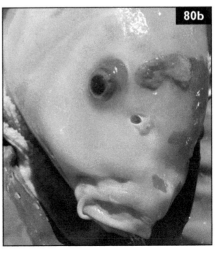

1 Without excess skin to create a primary closure, what is the expected course of healing for the mass removal site?
2 What is the prognosis for fish with a spindle cell neoplasm?
3 Why do you think the tumor recurred?

CASE 81 The aquarist noticed that several lionfish (*Pterois* sp.) in a mixed exhibit have red, swollen lumps on the tails, fins and around the mouth. The lesions have developed within the past week, the water quality is good, and all are eating and behaving normally. Skin and fin scrapes were non-remarkable.

1 What would you do next?
2 Should you revisit the history?

CASE 82 You identify the scale on a skin scraping (**82**) from an angelfish (*Pterophyllum* sp.).

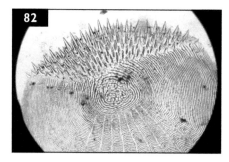

1 What type of scale is this?
2 Where does a scale arise in the skin (epidermis or dermis)?
3 Name other common types of scales and provide examples of species that have that type of scale.
4 How does the epidermis differ in fish without scales?

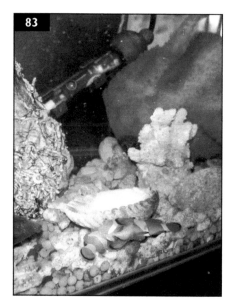

CASE 83 Two clownfish (*Amphiprion ocellaris*) housed in an aquarium with no history of disease or problems were found dead in the morning (**83**). They were fine when the owner retired for the evening.

1 What could have happened?
2 What gross signs can you observe to support the diagnosis?

CASE 84 A group of discus (*Symphysodon* sp.) are presented for anorexia, weight loss, abnormal appearing feces, and darkening of the skin. On necropsy examination the stomach wall is thickened. You perform a wet mount preparation of the stomach tissue (84).

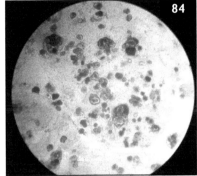

1 Identify the structures present in the stomach wall on wet mount examination.
2 What is the most likely causative agent?
3 Describe the organism's appearance on light microscopy.
4 What findings would you expect on histopathology of the internal organs?
5 What is required for definitive diagnosis?
6 What are the treatment options?

CASE 85

1 What would your differentials be for the lesions seen on this yellow perch (*Perca flavescens*) (85a)?
2 What diagnostic tests would you perform to arrive at a diagnosis?

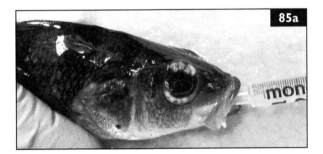

CASE 86 Anorexia is a non-specific clinical sign in captive elasmobranchs and may be the result of factors such as new environment, exhibit stressors, hormonal changes, diseases, etc. While it is important to understand the cause of the anorexia, regardless of the etiology, assist feeding is important to prevent dehydration, body weight loss, and malnutrition.

1 When is assist feeding indicated?
2 How can tube assist feeding be implemented and what should be fed?

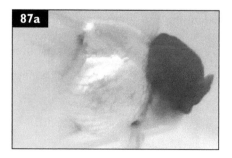

CASE 87 An oranda goldfish (*Carassius auratus*) is presented because its wen (head growth) has grown over the eyes and the fish is unable to see (87a).

1 How would you manage the situation?

CASE 88 The Murray cod (*Maccullochella peelii peelii*) is a large iconic freshwater fish found in Australia (88a). The fish in question was about 20 kg and had been in the public aquarium for 4–5 years in an 8,000 L (2,113 US gal) tank. It had a diminished appetite for several months, initially thought to be seasonal due to the lower winter water temperatures, but eventually it was decided to perform some diagnostic testing. The water level in the display was reduced by 70% and Aqui-S (commercial clove oil derivative) was added at 20 ppm to sedate the fish. A complete physical examination was performed, a blood sample collected from the caudal peduncle, and a gill sample taken. Fresh scrapes of the skin and fin were negative for parasites. The blood work appeared normal. The gill biopsy was placed in formalin and the histology photomicrograph is shown (88b).

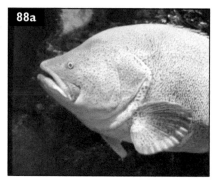

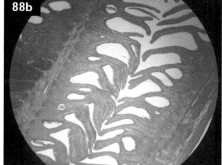

1 What is the problem?
2 What are the possible causes?

CASE 89 This is the lateral radiograph of a goldfish (*Carassius auratus*) taken under MS-222 anesthesia (**89**).

1 What are the two large radiolucent structures in the center of the image?
2 Are these normal?
3 How is radiography of this organ useful?

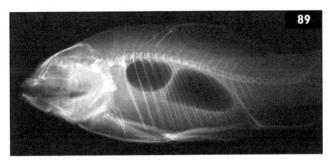

CASE 90 A 3-year-old, male, 173 g redcap oranda goldfish (*Carassius auratus*) presents with a chief complaint of anorexia lasting 2 days. The owners have observed the fish ('Goldie') staying primarily at the bottom of the water column and not showing his typical enthusiasm for food. The owners tell you Goldie will approach the food, occasionally ingest some, and then immediately regurgitate the pellets. During your initial examination of the unsedated fish in its clear, plastic travel container, you notice an area of inflammation ventrally along the lateral and medial aspects of the right mandible (**90a**). Your water quality testing and diagnostic wet mount cytology (gill biopsies and skin scrapes sampled from the sedated fish) are unremarkable.

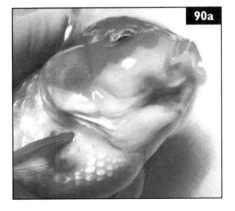

1 What questions would you like to ask the owners?
2 What else would you like to do?

CASE 91 A hobbyist in England has kept koi (*Cyprinus carpio*) in a 12,000 L (3,170 US gal) pond for over 20 years. Two weeks earlier he bought four small koi that had recently been imported from Japan and kept indoors in water at 19–20°C (66.2–68°F). Within a week of purchase, several of the hobbyist's original stock became lethargic, and lay on the bottom of the pond with their fins clamped against their body. They would roll onto their side for a few minutes, could still swim off when stimulated, and continued to eat well. A few koi floated upright near the surface or huddled in the corner of the pond near the water inlet. The problem had persisted for 10 days with no mortality and no response to a dose of flubendazole used to treat a suspected fluke infestation. Salt had been added to the pond and the salinity was 2.2 ppt. Water quality tests were within acceptable limits and the water temperature was 12–13°C (53.6–55.4°F). There were no obvious external lesions and no ectoparasites were found on several skin scrapes.

1 Suggest a course of action and possible diagnosis.

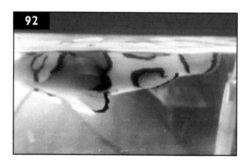

CASE 92 A newly purchased percula clownfish (*Amphiprion percula*) was treated for white spot disease (*Cryptocaryon* sp.) with copper sulfate in a hospital tank. Within minutes of application, the fish lost buoyancy control and floated to the surface (**92**).

1 Why is this, and how would you manage the situation?

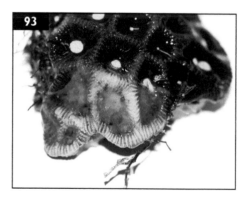

CASE 93

1 What abnormality can you identify on this piece of moon coral (*Favia* sp.) (**93**) and list various possible causes?

CASE 94 This 8-year-old oranda goldfish (*Carassius auratus*) was presented after floating at the surface with its right side uppermost for 2 weeks. The problem developed suddenly and there were no external lesions or known contributing factors. There is a slight asymmetrical swelling of the body. The fish was anesthetised with MS-222 and radiographs were taken (**94a, b**).

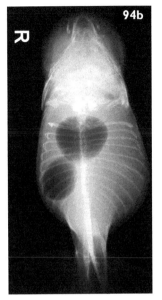

1 What abnormalities can be identified?
2 What is the most likely cause of the problem?
3 How can this be confirmed?
4 What treatment do you suggest?

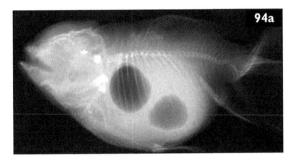

CASE 95 A 30 cm long, 6 kg, 10-year-old female koi (*Cyprinus carpio*) presents with a 5-day history of lethargy and anorexia. 'Sunshine,' a doitsu yamabuki ogon (a koi variety that is metallic yellow with very few scales), is housed in a 3,800 L (1,003 US gal) outdoor pond with six other koi that are now all normal per owner. The owner reports that 1 week ago all of the fish were behaving 'strangely,' staying on the bottom of the pond and not coming up to eat. This behavior only lasted a day before all fish except Sunshine returned to normal. Although the pond is relatively small for seven large koi, the life support system is adequate, and water quality parameters are within normal limits. All fish have been in the pond for 10 years and there have been no new additions. The owner thinks Sunshine also seems bloated.

As you are taking your history, you are also observing the fish in the pond. While the rest of the fish lazily swim about, you notice that Sunshine has isolated herself and is not moving very much. Her opercular movements are increased compared with the other fish. You do not observe any signs of flashing, piping, or gasping.

1 Is there significance to the sudden behavior change in all of the fish?
2 What are possible causes for an increased opercular rate (essentially an increased respiratory rate)?

CASE 96 You sedate the fish in **Case 95** with 75 ppm MS-222 (tricaine methanesulfonate). Irregular, superficial linear grooves that stretch the length of the body wall are noted on each side of the fish (**96a, b**). On the ventral aspect of the left operculum, you also notice an area of redness and superficial inflammation. Reflecting the operculum reveals an area of gill necrosis 2 × 2.5 cm. Her coelomic cavity is slightly distended but symmetrical. Overall, she demonstrates an increased body condition score (**96c**).

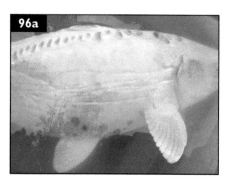

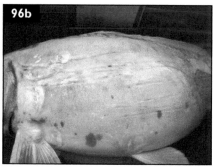

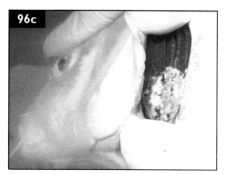

1 What is the most likely cause of these lesions?
2 How would you approach treatment?

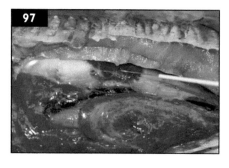

CASE 97

1 Name the structure pictured here (**97**) that is being sampled for bacterial culture and sensitivity in an adult koi (*Cyprinus carpio*).
2 Describe the physiologic function of this structure and how it differs from the other part of this organ.

CASE 98

1 What abnormality can you identify on this fragmented piece of pineapple coral (*Favia* sp.) (**98**)?
2 What effect does this have in marine reef systems?
3 How would this problem be controlled?

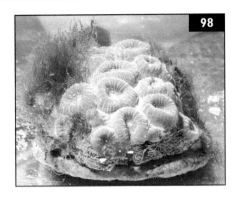

CASE 99 An emperor angelfish *(Pomacanthus imperator)* is scheduled to be treated for head and lateral line erosion (HLLE). While doing your physical examination you notice a large mass associated with the gills on one side (**99**) and several smaller masses on the other side (similar location).

1 What are your differential diagnoses?
2 What is your next step?

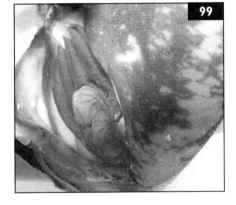

CASE 100 Some goldfish were reared as part of a research project to study the lifecycle of *Lernaea*. Normally, low numbers of *Lernaea* should not cause significant mortalities if conditions are good. Routine diagnostics found the fish were also infested with *Gyrodactylus* (**100**).

1 How would you manage this situation?

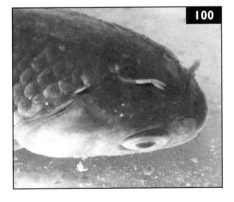

41

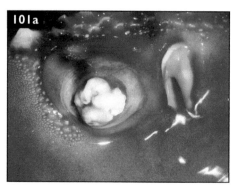

CASE 101 A juvenile bowmouth guitarfish (*Rhina ancylostoma*) was observed to have a cauliflower-like corneoconjunctival mass associated with the left eye (**101a**). The right eye looked good and the animal was feeding and behaving normally. The left eye was unaffected on arrival at the quarantine facility 1 month ago.

1 What causes would be included on your differential diagnosis list?
2 What diagnostic tests would you perform to determine the cause of the problem?
3 What is the cause of this lesion?

CASE 102 A bowmouth guitarfish (*Rhina ancylostoma*), also known as a 'shark ray,' had a sudden change to the appearance of one eye. There was no known trauma, or anything else in the history, that would explain this. When comparing both eyes, one could see that there was a difference (**102a, b**).

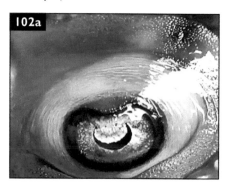
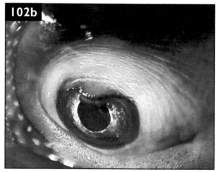

1 What is the name of the missing structure of the left eye (**102b**)?
2 What elasmobranchs have such a structure?
3 What is the purpose of this structure?
4 What might have happened and what would you do?

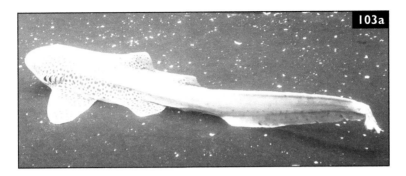

CASE 103 An adult, female zebra shark (*Stegostoma fasciatum*), which was housed in a 20,000,000 L (5,285,000 US gal) public aquarium system, was clinically observed to have a severely shredded tail tip. It was reported that an adult male zebra shark bit her tail during precopulatory behavior. She was behaving normally and in good body condition. The infected tail was observed to have a localized, 'moth-eaten', and shredded appearance with the underlying muscle and cartilage exposed (**103a**).

1 What is precopulatory behavior?
2 How would you treat this lesion?

CASE 104 A spotted moray eel (*Gymnothorax moringa*) developed a lump on its rostrum and was not eating (**104**). The other moray eels in the same exhibit were fine and the water quality was consistently good.

1 What is your recommendation for a next step?

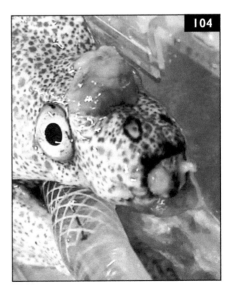

43

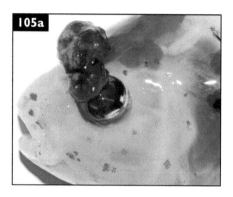
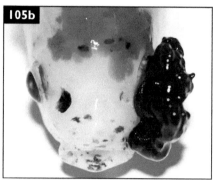

CASE 105 An 8-year-old comet-tailed goldfish (*Carassius auratus*) developed a mass on its left cornea that had been growing in size for a few weeks. Initially it occupied a third of the corneal surface and protruded significantly (**105a**). The mass was debulked and cauterized under anesthesia but an ultrasound scan revealed that it had infiltrated the corneal stroma and protruded into the anterior chamber of the eye. The fish recovered well but a few other small raised masses were noted on the body. Histologic examination identified the mass as a fibroma, a common neoplasm in goldfish. Over the following months the mass regrew and periodically fragments would break off. Five months after the initial surgery the mass was approximately twice the size of the globe (**105b**), although the fish continued to swim and eat normally. A further ultrasound scan revealed that the mass had invaded most of the globe.

1 Discuss the options available.

CASE 106 Prior to the removal of the eye from the fish in the **Case 105**, the educated owner had researched this procedure and found a scientific article that reported the fitting of a prosthesis to improve the appearance of these cases.

1 Discuss the practicality of such a cosmetic procedure.

CASE 107 The following questions deal with the important topic of biological filtration.

1 How would you describe biological filtration?
2 What can happen if a biological filter is not mature?
3 Can you give some examples of biological filter types?
4 What microorganisms are involved in biological filtration?

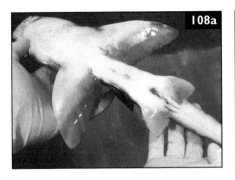
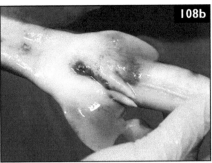

CASE 108 A juvenile zebra bullhead shark (*Heterodontus zebra*) was found lodged in the overflow of its 70,790 L (18,700 US gal) exhibit. Clinical manifestations include emaciation, dehydration, and reddish discoloration of the ventrum (**108a, b**). Blood was collected from the caudal vein and results showed leukocytosis. Clinical and laboratory findings strongly suggested septicemia.

1 What is the cause of these clinical signs?
2 How would you treat this case?

CASE 109 A female, juvenile Port Jackson shark (*Heterodontus portusjacksoni*) was observed with a localized, soft, round cyst measuring 13 mm in diameter on the right side of the perivent area (**109**). The rectal tract was normal and no prolapse was present.

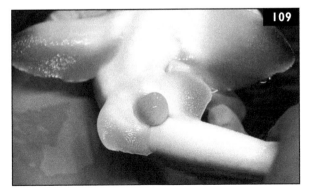

1 What is your diagnostic plan?
2 What might be the cause of this condition?
3 How would you manage this case?

45

CASE 110 A client with an established 17,100 L (4,500 US gal) pond with 18 adult koi (*Cyprinus carpio*) requests a pond call due to chronic problems in his

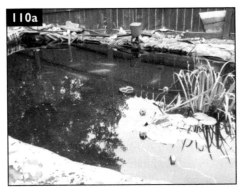

fish population including five deaths over the past winter. In addition, he has now observed red areas on several fish that also appear sluggish. On the phone, the client mentions he is upgrading the volume of the pond and adding additional filtration, but would like to determine the cause of these problems because he intends to add new fish once pond construction is complete.

On site (**110a**), you notice several bottom drains in the pond, a sand filter, an automatic feeder, and a high-end bead filtration system. Food pellets can be seen floating on the surface of the water. Koi food containers adjacent to the pond are in date and the food appears fresh. Several fish appear to have cutaneous ulcers and injected fins and tails. Two doitsu (scaleless) koi have reddened lateral lines. Occasional flashing by several koi is noted. A closer look at the flow through the filtration system shows the bottom drains and bead filter are currently offline, but the sand filter is in use. You choose two fish with representative lesions for sedation and closer examination. Skin scrapes are negative for parasites. Gill biopsies are also negative for parasites but the gill tissue appears hyperplastic. You note multiple areas of inflammation on the lateral line, fins, and tail of both fish examined. A few focal areas of ulceration are noted on the skin of both fish (**110b, c**).

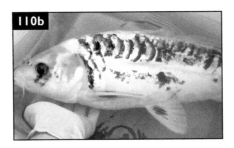
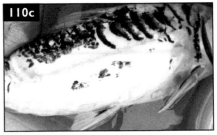

1 Is there anything in the history that may give a clue to the cause(s) of the current problem?
2 What is your next step?

CASE 111 A giant moray eel (*Gymnothorax javanicus*) apparently had a severe traumatic abdominal rupture. He was housed in a 43,060 L (11,375 US gal) public aquarium exhibit. Examination revealed a severe, irregularly-shaped avulsion located at the ventral mid-abdominal area exposing the underlying muscle layers, coelomic cavity, and some of the visceral organs (**111a**). Hemorrhage was not observed.

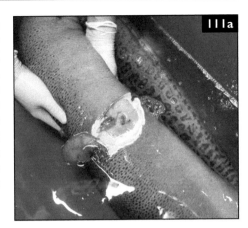

1 What was the likely cause of this wound?
2 How would you treat these lesions?
3 How could this condition be prevented?

CASE 112 A population of manta rays (*Manta* spp.) presented with multiple diffuse white patches on the skin and cephalic lobes (**112a**). They were housed in a 20,000,000 L (5,283,440 US gal) exhibit with mixed species of tropical fish and elasmobranchs. The system is supported by biological and mechanical filtration, ozone disinfection, and water temperature at 26–27°C (78.8–80.6°F). Standard water parameters are within normal limits.

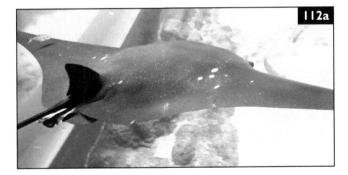

1 What would be your diagnostic plan?
2 How do caligoid copepods affect fish?
3 What is an appropriate treatment strategy?

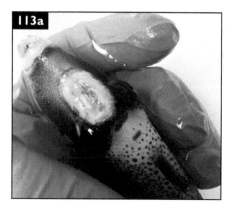

CASE 113 A 39 g, juvenile clown triggerfish (*Balistoides conspicillum*) presents with a 1 × 3 cm deep cutaneous ulcer between the eyes (**113a**). The lesion was first noticed 2 weeks prior to presentation. History reveals the owner successfully treated the fish with an over-the-counter product for a presumptive marine 'Ich' (*Cryptocaryon irritans*) infestation 3 weeks before the lesion appeared. Despite separate, prolonged immersion treatments of trimethoprim–sulfamethoxazole and ampicillin, the lesion progressed in size. Water quality tests are within normal limits and the diet and husbandry are excellent. The lesion is full thickness involving the skin and underlying structures. During the physical examination you note a central area of exposed dark tissue, resembling bone.

1 Are there any other questions you would like to ask?
2 What would be your next step?

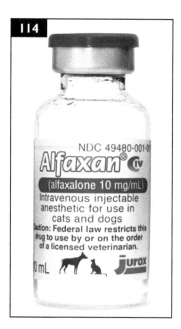

CASE 114 Alfaxalone has been used for anesthetizing fish (**114**).

1 What type of agent is alfaxalone?
2 How can it be applied to fish?
3 Is this compound approved for use in fish intended for human consumption?

CASE 115 An aquarist reports that a giant Pacific octopus (*Enteroctopus dofleini*) kept in a cold water exhibit has an abnormal growth on one arm. During observation, you note two irregularly-shaped masses located cranially between the mantle and arm, and another mass at the distal part of another arm. The masses are stretching the skin and floating away from the body. Close observation reveals multiple gas bubble accumulations in the subcutaneous layer (**115a, b**). The water quality parameters included temperature at 10.2°C (50.36°F), pH 7.84, salinity 30.59 ppt, and DO 114.3% (10.57 ppm).

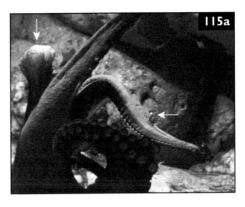

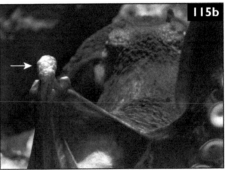

1 What is the cause of these clinical signs?
2 How would you treat this case?
3 How can this condition be prevented?

CASE 116 A farmer observes that 30% of tiger barbs (*Puntigrus tetrazona*) have moderate to severe ulcerative lesions of the rostrum and mouth several weeks after harvest from a pond. He submits four fish with zero to severe lesions to you for examination (**116a**). No significant findings are observed on wet mounts of the skin scrapings.

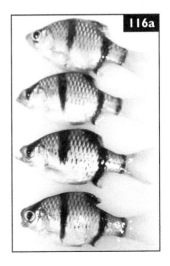

1 Based on these findings what should be at the top of your differential list?
2 How would you arrive at the diagnosis?

49

CASE 117 A pet store that has been in business for over 10 years is losing wild-caught *Corydoras*, cardinal tetras (*Paracheirodon axelrodi*), and blue rams (*Mikrogeophagus ramirezi*) in one of their freshwater systems soon after arrival from the primary supplier. Scats (*Scatophagus argus*), archerfish (*Toxotes* sp.), and Colombian sharks (*Sciades seemani*) are not affected. Fish appear normal on receipt but die after 2–5 days. No clinical signs are apparent on receipt and only some lethargy and water column 'hanging' is observed prior to death. This problem has been ongoing for three shipments over 8 weeks. The owner also mentions that (1) they have not seen any signs of flashing, external parasites, or had an 'Ich' outbreak in a few months and (2) they have not been able to keep any plants alive for a while in the affected system. Three days post-shipment you check the water quality parameters and find total ammonia nitrogen 0, nitrite 0, pH 6.5, temperature 25°C (77°F), DO 6.5 mg/L, alkalinity 51 mg/L $CaCO_3$, hardness 205 mg/L. Skin, fin, and gill samples from representative moribund fish of all species are negative for parasites.

1 What questions would you like to ask the owners?
2 What additional diagnostic tests would you recommend?

CASE 118 Referring to **Case 117**:

1 Are any of the water quality parameters provided of additional concern in the pet store's system?
2 What additional water quality data would be necessary for a more complete picture of the system?

CASE 119 A newly purchased group of oscars (*Astronotus ocellatus*) exhibits anorexia, depression, and huddling at the bottom of a pet store's tank. Circular structures filled with small dot-like organisms are seen on gill biopsy (**119a**).

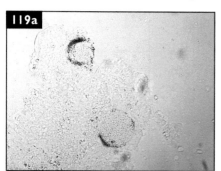

1 What is the cause of the lesions and how would you treat this condition?

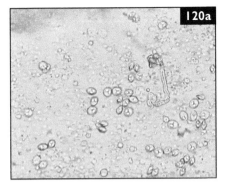

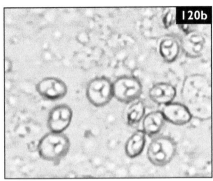

CASE 120 An aquarium fish wholesaler recently imported bala sharks (also known as tricolor shark minnows, *Balantiocheilos melanopterus*) from Thailand. After 1 week, chronic mortalities began to occur. Affected fish appeared to hang in the water column, lose condition, and demonstrate abnormal swimming/darting behaviors. Bacterial cultures of brain and kidney on standard blood agar (tryptic soy agar with sheep's blood) were negative at 28°C (82.4°F) after 48 hours. The only wet mount lesions seen were from the brain (**120a, b**; low-power and high-power magnification, respectively).

1 What are these structures?
2 What would you recommend to the wholesaler?

CASE 121 A transhipper of tropical fish asks you to examine a tank of moribund opaline gourami (*Trichopodus trichopterus*). Some fish present with an enlarged coelom. You select them for euthanasia and necropsy, and observe the organisms shown in the intestinal contents (**121a**).

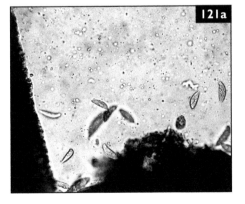

1 What are these organisms?
2 Do you recommend treating for this condition?

51

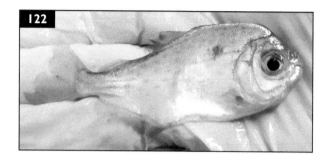

CASE 122 A knowledgeable client makes an appointment to see you because of chronic frayed fin problems with her mixed-species South American freshwater aquarium. She has not added any new fish in over a year, there has been no mortality, and the pet store found the pH, ammonia, nitrite, chlorine, and DO levels all within normal limits. Today she brings you a 1 L water sample and a silver dollar fish (*Metynnis* sp.) with tattered caudal, dorsal, and anal fins (122). She also reports that her filtration is so good these days, with a combination of mechanical, biological and chemical filtration, that she rarely does water changes. She also emphasizes that she is purely a fish person and the only plants in her aquarium are made of plastic.

1 How would you approach this case?
2 What recommendations will you have for this client?

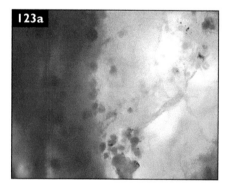

CASE 123 A hobbyist who specializes in breeding discus (*Symphysodon* spp.) informs you that some appear thin despite having a good appetite. He has also noted a decrease in productivity. Occasionally a fish dies despite treatment with metronidazole. He submits a moribund discus for examination. You see numerous structures (123a) in the stomach and upper intestine.

1 What are they and what is the likely cause?
2 How would you manage this problem?

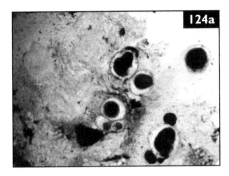
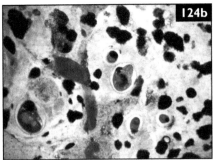

CASE 124 A group of several hundred grunts (*Haemulon* sp.) held at a quarantine facility for several weeks prior to display at a public aquarium have begun to experience chronic mortalities. The dead fish (morts) were in good condition prior to death and died acutely. The primary findings, and consistently identified squash preparation lesions, are shown (**124a, b**).

1 What is this tissue (most likely) and what are the primary lesions?
2 Bench top stains and histology were negative for acid-fast bacteria. What might explain this? What other bacterial disease should be high on the differential list and what additional diagnostics would be required?

CASE 125 With regard to the grunts in **Case 124**:

1 What would your recommendation be to this public aquarium?

CASE 126 On reviewing histologic slides of a *Corydoras* catfish, you observe bilateral glandular structures near the 'shoulder' of the fish (**126**).

1 What are these structures?

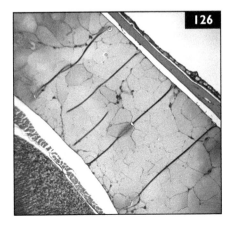

53

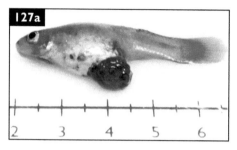

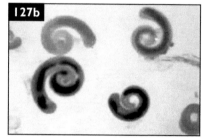

CASE 127 A pond of 10,000 swordtails (*Xiphophorus hellerii*) is harvested by an aquarium fish producer in Florida and all fish are behaving and swimming normally and eating well. However, approximately 20% appear to have mild to moderate coelomic distension, and 5% have severe coelomic distension (**127a**). Microscopic evaluation of wet mounts of coelomic masses revealed curled structures (**127b**).

1 What are these structures?
2 What management options would you recommend to the producer?

CASE 128 A koi (*Cyprinus carpio*) wholesaler has had disease issues with international fish imported to his facility in the spring (system temperature, 24°C [75.2°F]) and domestic koi arriving in summer (system temperature 28°C [82.4°F]). A large percentage of the fish in both groups, either immediately on arrival, or soon after, would lie on the bottom immobile (**128a, b**), but would swim up for food or respond when the tank was struck. Some fish appeared to have pale swollen gills and enophthalmia. Both groups experienced ongoing low level mortalities.

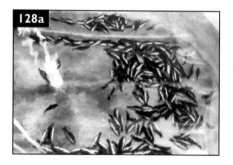

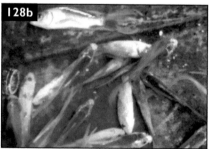

1 What additional information do you need?
2 What are some differential diagnoses and how would you rule these out?

CASE 129 A new koi (*Cyprinus carpio*) producer is having problems with a large percentage of his grow-outs. The fish are generally eating well and have no behavioral abnormalities. Two koi (both to be culled for poor coloration) from his facility are pictured (**129**). The fish are being raised in clear ponds with poor productivity (no phytoplankton growth, very low alkalinity, but moderate hardness) and are being fed a standard tilapia diet.

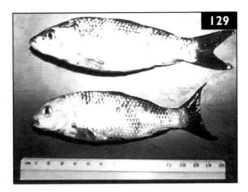

1 Which koi is abnormal, and why?
2 Given the history, what are some probable causes for this abnormality and what would be your management recommendations?

CASE 130 A group of yoyo loaches (*Botia almorhae*) present with a gray sheen on their skin. A skin scraping and gill biopsy reveal numerous small translucent motile protists, some of which are attached to skin and gill (**130a**, arrows).

1 What are these protists?
2 How would you treat this condition?

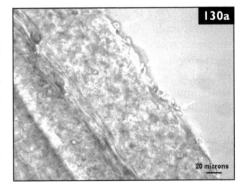

CASE 131 Your practice is located in a southern US city that has recently experienced an unusual ice storm, which has led to widespread power outages and persistent sub-freezing temperatures. The local television station has asked you to come on the air and address the crisis with regard to aquarium pets.

1 What recommendations can you make with regard to the following parameters: food, temperature, water quality, and lighting?

55

CASE 132 A busy fourth year medical student from a nearby university makes an appointment to see you about her 5-year-old pet tilapia (*Oreochromis mossambicus*) (132). The fish lives alone (and always has) since the owner

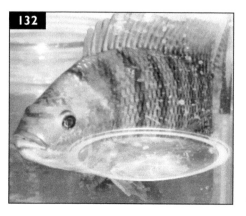

adopted it from a college vertebrate zoology laboratory 4 years prior. The fish has acclimated quite well to a 110 L (29 US gal) aquarium that is heated, lighted, and filtered with a large canister filter. The presenting complaint is the fish is listless and stopped eating about 3 days ago. While taking the history you learn that the owner normally changes 30% of the water each month with dechlorinated tap water. They accomplish this with a python siphon apparatus and clean the 5 cm of gravel substrate at the same time. You also learn the student was recently in South America for 3 months as part of a medical charity effort. While away she had a friend feeding the fish but not doing water changes. When your client returned from her trip the fish looked great so she was not worried about the water quality. In addition, she was starting a busy emergency rotation at the local hospital and had very little time at home for the next 8 weeks. It was near the end of this rotation that she noticed her fish did not look right. You test the water and find the following: ammonia 2.5 ppm; nitrite 0.05 ppm; nitrate 5.0 ppm; alkalinity 40 ppm; hardness 50 ppm; pH 4.5.

1 How can you account for these results?
2 What are your recommendations?

CASE 133 The local tropical fish club has asked you to give a talk on emergency care and support of pet fish in the home in the absence of, or pending, veterinary care. Your talk is focused on topics such as power outages, chlorine and other toxic events (e.g. pesticides), leaky or broken aquaria, trauma, and fish jumping out of aquaria. Your presentation is well received and there is a request for a list of supplies to be kept in a pet fish emergency preparedness box.

1 What items would you include on such a list?

CASE 134 An adult koi (*Cyprinus carpio*) weighing 662 g presents for a 2-week history of floating left side down. The owners have had the fish for about 1 year and obtained it from a friend. For the past 10 days the fish has been isolated in a tub of pond water with some kosher salt. The koi did not improve so a couple of ampicillin capsules were added to the tub; there was still no improvement.

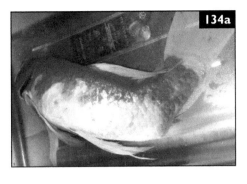

When you examine the fish you note the fish is indeed positively buoyant with its left side up. The fish is moderately curved and the concave (right) side of the body is hyperemic. The caudal peduncle and caudal fin are flexed dorsally (**134a**).

1 What questions would you like to ask the owners?
2 What diagnostic tests would you recommend?

CASE 135 Regarding **Case 134**:

1 Why was the question about electrical storms included with the history taking?

CASE 136 An adult electric eel (*Electrophorus electricus*) weighing 18 kg and measuring 2 m in length presents acutely. A large metal screw protrudes through its ventrolateral body wall about 30 cm caudal to the mouth (**136a**). The visible part of the screw is approximately 15 cm long. The animal has been anorexic for 4 days. The fish belongs to a zoo and is kept in a display aquarium.

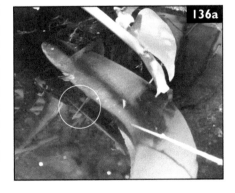

1 What concerns do you have when handling electric eels?
2 What diagnostic tests would you recommend?
3 How would you perform anesthesia in this case? How would you assess depth of anesthesia during induction?

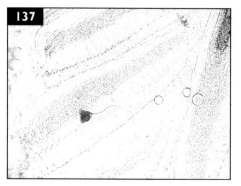

CASE 137 The owner of a fish store reports that some marine fish have skin lesions. As an example he presents a tang (*Acanthurus* sp.) with a pale area just below the dorsal fin. You scrape the area and examine it as a wet mount with a light microscope and see this (**137**).

1 What is this organism?
2 Would you recommend treatment, and if so, with what?

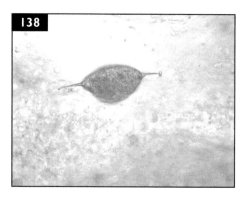

CASE 138 You find this structure (**138**) on a gill biopsy of the fish in Case 137.

1 What is this structure?

CASE 139 You have been summoned to act as a liaison between a koi (*Cyprinus carpio*) farm client, the state veterinarian, and the US Department of Agriculture (USDA) Animal, Plant, Health Inspection Service (APHIS) veterinarian related to a suspected outbreak of spring viremia of carp virus (SVCv).

1 Provide a summary of SVCv.
2 What are your obligations as a licensed USDA APHIS accredited veterinarian when dealing with a suspected case?
3 How would you proceed to collect and submit samples?
4 What type of legal follow-up is required for affected facilities?

CASE 140 In mid-October you are called out to see a North Carolina koi (*Cyprinus carpio*) pond where there has been recent morbidity and mortality. The 18 koi were living in the pond when the current homeowners purchased the house and property about 1 year ago. According to a neighbor, the fish may have been in the pond for 10 years. At one time the pond held as many as 40 fish but some of these were sold.

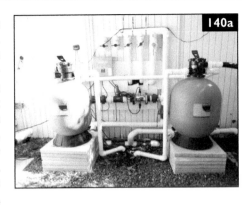

One fish died last winter and a second in June. Three fish perished over the last 2 days. The 52,000 L (13,736 gallon) rubber-lined pond was completely rebuilt within the last year by a professional aquatic systems company. The life support system includes two bottom drains, a skimmer, waterfall, paired pumps, advanced biological filtration, and a twin 400W UV filtration unit (**140a**). The water turns over every 60–90 minutes with minimal water current being generated. The feeding protocol for the pond is appropriate. There have been no recent additions to the population. There is a laterally recumbent moribund fish in the skimmer that will be easy to capture and examine.

1 What are your next steps?

CASE 141 A juvenile striped burrfish (*Chilomycterus schoepfi*) presented with a several week history of coelomic distension. It is housed in a mixed-species brackishwater exhibit designed to replicate a salt marsh. The fish is reported to be eating well and behaving normally. When removed from the water and held in dorsal recumbency for physical examination, the distension resolves (**141a**).

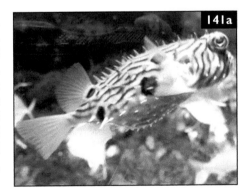

1 What diagnostic procedures can be performed to diagnose the cause of coelomic distension?
2 What considerations in the exhibit and husbandry might be taken to reduce the incidence of this condition?

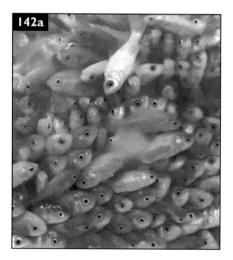

CASE 142 A pet store recently purchased 1,000 comets (*Carassius auratus*) and reports the fish are sluggish and lying on the bottom of the tank. Mortality has been low and fish will resume normal position and swim in response to stimulation; however, they return to the bottom afterwards. On a visit to the store you observe they tend to group tightly together (**142a**). The tank is more than large enough for the stocking density. You collect several moribund comets for examination and observe numerous irregular structures in the intestine (**142b**, arrows).

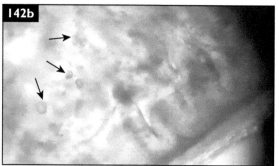

1 How could you further pursue diagnostics in this case?

CASE 143 A new client approaches you about a wellness examination for their newly purchased aquarium and its inhabitants. They obtained the large aquarium as part of the deal with a recent home purchase. They are not experienced hobbyists and have no idea of the size (volume) of the tank. They know it is 'big,' rectangular, and contains an assortment of South American cichlids and catfish. As part of the telephone history your receptionist would like to know the volume of the aquarium.

1 What measurements should your receptionist request from the client in order to accurately determine the volume and what equation would you use?
2 If this were a cylindrical aquarium, what measurements would you need and in what equation?

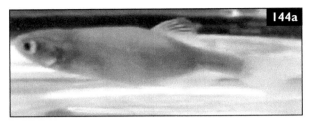

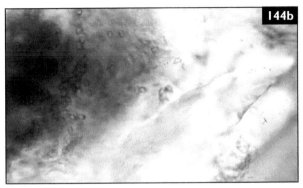

CASE 144 A client complains that one of her danios (zebrafish) (*Danio rerio*) has become very pale (**144a**). On gross examination you observe the dorsal epaxial muscles are bulging on the left side. There are no significant findings on routine wet mount examination of external tissues. You recommend euthanasia and necropsy. A wet mount of the muscle tissue is shown (**144b**).

1 What is the likely cause of the problem?

CASE 145 You are a consultant for a local science museum that has a number of aquatic systems. One is a trout exhibit with a large open area that affords close access by the public. In addition to 10 brook trout (*Salvelinus fontinalis*) there are some cold-water cyprinids and yellow perch (*Perca flavescens*). The curator reports that two of the trout have been off feed for about 1 week and seem lethargic. All of the other fish in the system appear normal and a recent and thorough water quality screen revealed no abnormalities. While taking the history you learn that a trout died about a month ago and is in the museum's freezer.

1 What is your diagnostic plan?
2 What are your recommendations?

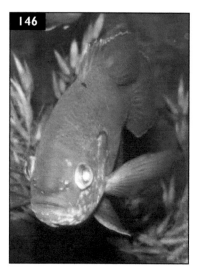

CASE 146 A 5-year-old dollar sunfish (*Lepomis marginatus*) presents for evaluation of a unilateral cataract. The fish is a collection animal at a local museum and the cataract was first noticed by the keeper staff approximately 6 months ago. Physical examination reveals a mature cataract and a partial anterior lens luxation in the left eye (**146**). The remainder of the examination is unremarkable.

1 What additional history questions are important in this case?
2 What diagnostic tests are indicated?
3 What management options will you propose for this animal?

CASE 147 With regard to **Case 146**, the decision was made to surgically remove the cataract. Phacoemulsification was successful for the lens cortex but the nucleus was too compact for this technique.

1 How would you manage this challenge?
2 How would you manage this case after surgery?

CASE 148 Pictured is an image of a blood film from a bullnosed ray (*Myliobatis freminvillii*) (**148**).

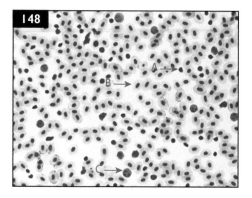

1 Name the cells indicated by the letters and arrows.

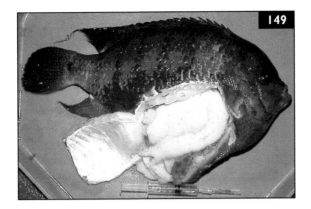

CASE 149 A large, mature Pearsei cichlid (*Cichlasoma pearsei*) dies after a prolonged illness, and you perform a necropsy (**149**).

1 What immediately strikes you as abnormal about the *in-situ* visceral cavity?
2 How can you quickly confirm the constitution of the large white mass?
3 What may have led to this condition?

CASE 150 A pet store recently purchased a group of young keyhole cichlids (*Cleithracara maronii*). The owner reports approximately 50% of them have an enlarged eye (**150a**). You observe the fish and note that some fish have a unilateral cataract (**150b**), some have unilateral pupillary miosis, and some have unilateral exophthalmia. Despite this, the fish are feeding and acting normally.

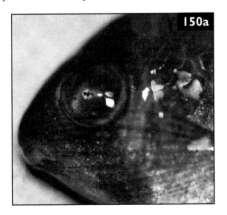
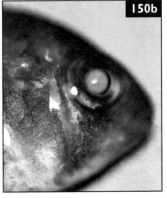

1 What do you suspect and how will you confirm your suspicion?

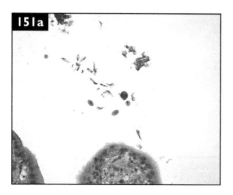

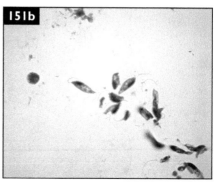

CASE 151 A hobbyist recently purchased a group of angelfish (*Pterophyllum scalare*). Some of the fish have distended coeloms and are listless. At necropsy you observe rapidly swimming flagellated organisms in the lumen of the intestine (**151a, b** [approximately 100× and 400× magnification respectively]).

1 What do you suspect?

CASE 152 A hobbyist purchased a group of *Corydoras* catfish, and several days after purchase they began to exhibit anorexia and decreased activity. On gross examination, you observe gray and creamy patches on the dorsum of the fish. You perform a scraping of one of the patches and observe certain features at 400× magnification (**152a**). The organisms are shown in an H&E-stained histologic photomicrograph (**152b**, arrow).

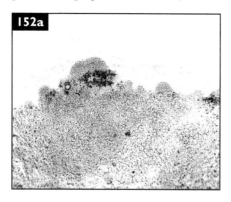

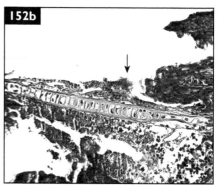

1 What is this condition?
2 What treatment do you recommend?

CASE 153 An ornamental fish farmer complains that he has been losing zebra danios (*Danio rerio*) within his ponds and vat rooms. He explains that it appears worse in the spring and fall months. The fish exhibit exophthalmia along with hemorrhage in the skin around the eyes, cranium (hole-in-the-head), operculum, base of the fins, and abdomen (**153a**). Additionally, they have swollen abdomens due to ascites (**153b**) and they display neurologic swimming behaviors such as spinning, spiraling, and lethargy (**153c**). Water quality is within normal limits for the species and external biopsies are unremarkable.

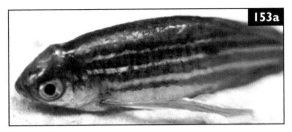

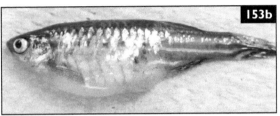

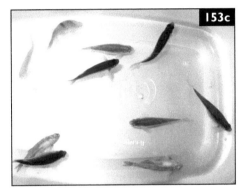

1 What further diagnostics should be performed?
2 What is the diagnosis?

CASE 154

1 Identify this parasite (**154a**) that was found in the small intestine of a fish on the necropsy floor.
2 How does this parasite feed? Briefly discuss its life cycle.
3 If you were to treat this condition, how would you accomplish this?

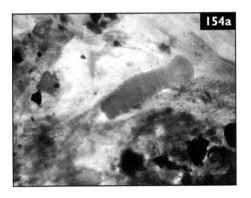

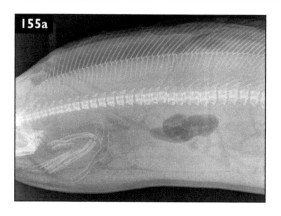
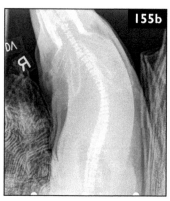

CASE 155 An adult green moray eel was found acutely lethargic, in lateral recumbency, with abnormally rapid gulping motions of the mouth (increased respiratory rate) and superficial wounds to the tail due to aggression from tank mates. The eel was anesthetized with immersion in tricaine methanesulfonate (MS-222) for diagnostic radiographs (155a, b).

1 What lesion(s) are evident in these images?
2 What is a possible etiology for this injury?

CASE 156 You make a field call to evaluate a 12-year-old female goldfish (*Carassius auratus*) for coelomic distension and cutaneous edema ('pineconing') of

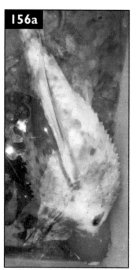

1 week's duration. It is November and this fish is housed outdoors with 10 other goldfish who are all doing well in a 3,800 L (1,000 US gal) pond. Physical examination reveals symmetrical, moderate-severe coelomic distension and moderate cutaneous edema (156a, b).

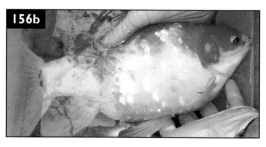

1 What diagnostic tests are indicated?
2 What is the prognosis?

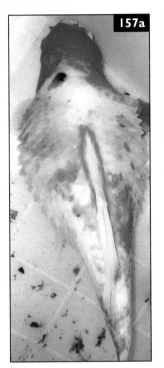

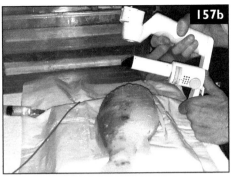

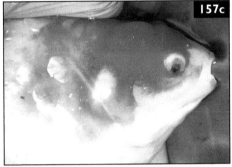

CASE 157 With regard to **Case 156**, medicated baths were performed for 6 weeks and then discontinued by the owner. The fish's coelomic distension worsened during this time but it continued to eat. Once the medicated baths were discontinued, the fish stopped eating, and became more lethargic. The goldfish presented to your clinic for a recheck 2 months after the initial examination (**157a**). Physical examination revealed worsening coelomic distension, persistent cutaneous edema, and multifocal cutaneous erythema.

1 What diagnostic tests are indicated?
2 What treatment options will you recommend?
3 What is the prognosis?
  Six weeks later, the fish presented for evaluation of unilateral ocular trauma. Her coelom remained distended, the cutaneous edema was still present, and her cutaneous erythema had progressed. Consultation with a veterinary ophthalmologist confirmed a deep corneal ulcer, but revealed the globe to be intact (**157b, c**).
4 What other diagnostic tests are indicated?
5 What treatments are recommended?

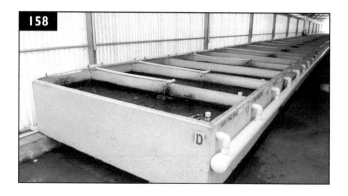

CASE 158 An aquaculture farmer complains that within three separate recirculating aquaculture systems on his farm he notices the fish are exhibiting signs of lethargy, have increased respiratory rates, and there is a spike in cases of columnaris disease and mortality. He mentions that every week vats (**158**) within the systems are taken off line and sterilized with calcium hypochlorite bleaching powder for a minimum of 1 hour. The vats are neutralized with sodium thiosulfate, drained, scrubbed cleaned, rinsed, and placed back on the system before being refilled with system water as fish are sold and replaced with new stock. Until 3 weeks ago the weekly water quality parameter readings had been unremarkable. The current water quality parameters are: temperature 27–29°C (80.6–84.2°F); ammonia 2.8–3.4 mg/L; nitrite 0 mg/L; pH 8.0–8.4; total hardness 225–250 mg/L; total alkalinity 200–240 mg/L ($CaCO_3$). During your history you learn that workers had been using decreasing amounts of sodium thiosulfate while they awaited the purchase of a new 20 kg bag.

1 What is the probable diagnosis and cause?
2 How would you manage this situation?

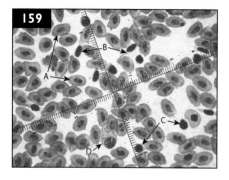

CASE 159 Pictured is an image of a blood film from a hybrid striped bass (*Morone chrysops x M. saxatilis*) (**159**).

1 Name the cells indicated by the letters and arrows.

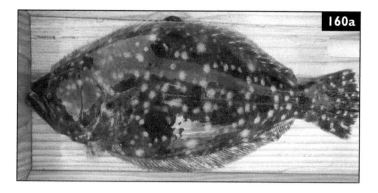

160a

CASE 160 A cohort of 10 broodstock southern flounder (*Paralicthys lethostigma*) is being kept in a low salinity environment to test the suitability of that approach for aquaculture production (**160a**). Southern flounder are euryhaline fish that adapt to fresh and marine water at different life stages, making them a suitable candidate for culture in low salinity environments. On necropsy of an individual from the same cohort for unrelated purposes, there was an incidental finding of 100% calcium hydrogen phosphate dehydrate (brushite) urinary bladder stones. The broodstock are kept in a 4,950 L (1,307 US gal) closed system with salinity 1.25 ppt (min 0.9, max 1.46), total hardness 140.91 grains per gallon (gpg) (min 90, max 190), calcium hardness 100.91 gpg (min 70, max 160), magnesium hardness 40 gpg (max 30, max 50). The remaining water quality parameters are unremarkable and considered within normal limits.

1 How would you proceed?
2 What diagnostic imaging may help diagnose urinary bladder stones?

CASE 161 With regard to **Case 160**:

1 What possible etiologies may be playing an underlying role in this disease presentation?

CASE 162 You have been asked to present a lecture on medicating pet fish to a group of veterinary students.

1 Review appropriate injection sites applicable to most fish.
2 Discuss why the subcutaneous route is not commonly used.

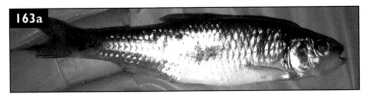

163a

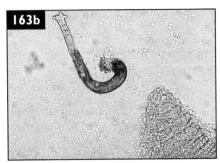

163b

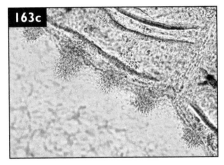

163c

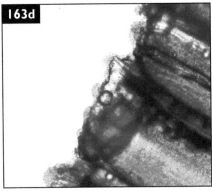

163d

CASE 163 A representative sample of shiner minnows (*Notropis* sp.) from a laboratory system present for sudden and acute system collapse described as 70% mortality. The housing tank is a recirculating system with adequate filtration, water quality parameters within acceptable limits, and no previous problems. The shiners were collected 3 days prior to the mortality event using a seine at a local creek and acclimated prior to introduction to the system, although no quarantine period or treatments were completed. External examination of the affected fish revealed mild erythema along the ventrum, caudal and anal fins, and a frayed dorsal fin. The gills revealed no gross lesions. The remaining physical examination of both live and recently deceased fish revealed no remarkable findings (163a). Skin scrapes and gill clips are collected and evaluated at 40× magnification. The initial microscopic evaluation reveals a single monogenean, *Dactylogyrus* sp. (163b). Delayed review (15 minutes following biopsy procurement) of the slides reveals clumped masses ('haystacks') of writhing, long, thin bacterial rods on the periphery of the skin (163c) and fin (163d) biopsies in large numbers.

1 What disease are these findings highly suggestive of?
2 What treatment protocol would you suggest and what recommendations would you make prior to restocking the system?

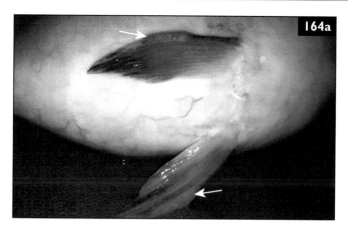

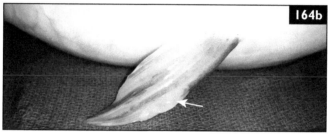

CASE 164 A koi (*Cyprinus carpio*) client contacts you in late spring complaining of what he believes to be pink to pale, raised and smooth lesions on the fins and skin of several koi in his 15,000 L (3,962 US gal) pond (**164a, b,** arrows). The fish are eating and behaving normally. There has been no mortality and the water tests are completely normal on the owner's test kit. The water temperature is 15°C (59° F). Notable in the history is that the owner added four new koi the previous summer after an inadequate quarantine period.

1 What disease is at the top of your differential list?
2 What conditions should also be considered?
3 How can you confirm the diagnosis?
4 How will you manage the problem?

CASE 165

1 What is a sponge filter and how does it function?
2 How can sponge filters be employed to increase biosecurity?

CASE 166 The large public aquarium where you work has a satellite holding facility. Late on a Friday afternoon one of the administrators is not happy with the color of the water in two large shark tanks (actually above ground swimming pools) that contain seven brown shark (*Carcharhinus plumbeus*) pups. The issue is that some potential donors will be touring the facility in the upcoming week. The biggest concern is yellow looking water caused by a build-up of dissolved organic carbon (DOC). The carbon comes directly from uneaten food and animal waste. Other than appearance, DOC is not a big problem for the short term, and it can be managed in several ways.

Several aquarists were instructed to put an inline carbon filter on the two pools. The shark pups had been collected earlier that summer. They were doing quite well, eating a lot, and growing. The simple systems were composed of 3.7 m diameter swimming pools with a suction intake to a pump. Out of the pump the water flow was split, with one portion returning directly to the tank, below the surface, and the remainder to a slow bio/sand filter. From the filter the water tumbled back into the shark holding pools. The tumbling action entrained lots of air, creating a constant column of bubbles in the holding tank. That air–water interface kept the DO levels above 90% in the pools.

That afternoon the already stretched thin aquarists were exhausted from a week of collecting, moving animals, and facility construction. Despite their best efforts and last minute planning they did not have the parts for the inline filters. The supervisor made the decision to add a porous bag containing 1 kg (2.2 lb) of activated carbon into the pipe returning water to one pool. This way all water would have to contact the carbon before returning to the pool. Everything went well except the carbon bag impeded the flow enough that the water would back up into the bio/sand filter and begin to overflow. After changing some valve positions, the staff watched for a few minutes and determined everything was running well. The shark pups were swimming fine when the staff left. Unfortunately, they were found dead the next morning. The sharks in the other pool, where no modifications occurred, were normal and healthy.

1 What would be on your differential list for the cause of death?
2 How could you make the diagnosis?
3 How could the DOC accumulation be managed better and safer?

CASE 167

1 What is UV filtration and how does it work?
2 What are some disadvantages and limitations of this technology?

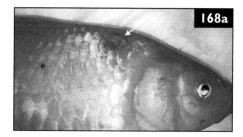

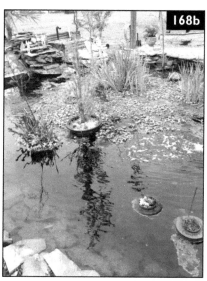

CASE 168 Three deceased young adult koi (*Cyprinus carpio*) present for evaluation of mild skin ulcers (168a, arrow), abnormal behavior, and mortality. These fish represent about 20 other fish that were kept in the same 18,900 L (5,000 US gal) outdoor koi pond (168b). The pond has historically been continuously fed by well water and continuously drained via an overflow, although about 3 weeks ago the water source was cut off.

The koi have a 2-year history of developing skin ulcers, which are worse in the summer. When they develop ulcers they are treated with malathion (Spectracide®, 50% malathion), as advised by an employee at the koi store, and the sores improve. The treatment protocol is 1 oz diluted (30 ml) in water and added to the pond, a rest day, then 1.5 oz followed by a rest day, then 3 oz.

It is late March and recently the koi started to develop skin ulcers again. Malathion treatment was initiated and the fish started to display erratic swimming (circling), jumping out of the water, and floating on the surface on their sides. Three days after initiating treatment five fish died acutely and over the next 48 hours all of the other fish in the pond died.

1 Calculate the level of malathion present in the pond.
2 What testing could be pursued to confirm your diagnosis?

CASE 169 A 33.3 kg goliath grouper (*Epinenphelus itajara*) ingested a rectangular plastic water sampling bottle, approximately 14 × 10 × 4 cm, aggressively grasped from the hand of an aquarist collecting the sample.

1 What potential outcomes could result from this ingestion?
2 What diagnostics and/or interventions might be necessary to ensure the well-being of this fish?

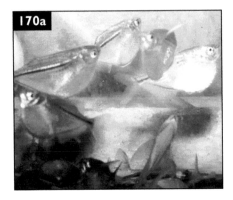

170a

CASE 170 A pet store contacts you because they are experiencing high mortality in a tank of silver hatchetfish (*Gasteropelicus sternicla*) (**170a**). The fish were purchased from a wholesaler 5 days prior and have been kept in an isolated system. Most of the surviving fish have labored respiration and appear weak and disoriented. The fish room manager has tried immersion treatment with tetracycline and Melafix® without success. The water tests normal and the rest of the aquaria in the facility look good. Skin biopsies are unremarkable but the gills are covered with numerous heart-shaped ciliated structures (approximately 30–50 μm in length) that move in a slow, circular pattern when not on the gill tissue (**170b**).

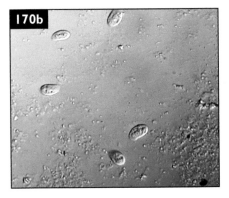

170b

1 What is the most likely diagnosis?
2 Why have the over the counter treatments (OTC) treatments been unrewarding?
3 How would you manage this case?

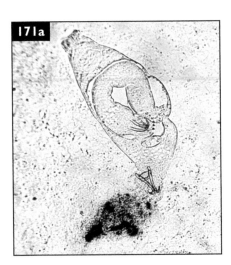

171a

CASE 171 The organism pictured (**171a**) was found on a gill biopsy from a koi (*Cyprinus carpio*) in a large pond on a routine health screening. The 20,000 L (5,284 US gal) pond contains about a dozen mature fish between 1 and 3 kg and all appear clinically normal.

1 What type of organism is this and briefly review its natural history?
2 Can you identify it by taxonomic family, and if so, how?
3 Would you institute therapy, and if so, what regimen would you choose?

CASE 172 An ornamental aquaculture farmer notes that he consistently has chronic low-level mortality with the sunset variatus platies (*Xiphophorus* sp.) that he receives from a local vendor. Numerous attempts at bacterial isolation via culture of the brain and posterior kidney have been unrewarding. External biopsies are negative for parasites, but long flexing bacterial rods that clump together to form haystacks are noted on the skin scrape and fin clip. *Flavobacterium columnare*, the causative agent of columnaris disease, has caused recurring infections in which treatment clears the infection, but the platies inevitably become reinfected. Columnaris disease commonly occurs when fish are stressed and immunocompromised. The water parameters are within normal limits for the species and external biopsies and brain and posterior kidney cultures are negative, therefore samples are submitted for histopathology to rule out other causes.

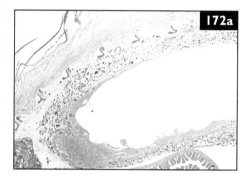

1 In **172a** what is the structure and what are the organisms seen within and around it?
2 What is your diagnosis and recommendation?

CASE 173 A newly acquired rainbow trout (*Oncorhynchus mykiss*) is found to have three macroscopic organisms attached to its caudal fin (**173**). As the consulting veterinarian for a large outdoor provisions store with large coldwater and temperate systems, you are asked to identify these organisms and advise the aquarist on a management strategy. Fortunately the fish is still in quarantine and isolated.

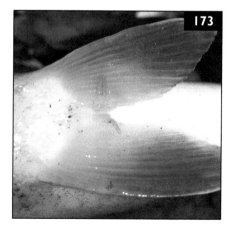

1 What are these organisms?
2 How would you manage this issue?

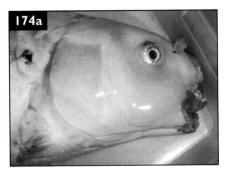

CASE 174 An owner discovers several koi (*Cyprinus carpio*) scattered around her pond, mutilated and half eaten. The pond is located on her property in the Sandhills region of North Carolina, surrounded by pine forests and many natural and man-made bodies of water. Affected fish exhibit trauma primarily to their heads and fins. In spite of severe injuries to its face and missing fins, one 3.6 kg 6-year-old male koi is still moving and able to be revived (**174a**). The client calls you out to investigate the incident and examine this fish.

1 What koi pond predator(s) are known to cause this sort of damage?
2 The client wants to know if this koi can be saved and asks you whether or not it should it be euthanized?
3 How would you treat and rehabilitate this fish?

CASE 175 A pet store contacts you because they are experiencing high morbidity and mortality in a tank of blue damselfish (*Chrysiptera cyanea*). The fish were purchased from a wholesaler 1 week prior and have been kept on an isolated

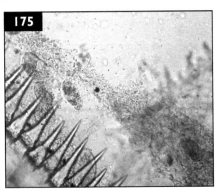

system. Some of the fish have areas of depigmentation and mild hyperemia and many fish appear to have labored respiration. The fish room manager has tried a number of over the counter (OTC) antibiotics without success. You test the water and it is within normal limits. Gill and skin biopsies reveal numerous heart-shaped structures (approximately 50 μm long) gliding over the epithelial tissues or moving in a slow circular motion when not on the surface of the fish (**175**).

1 What is the most likely diagnosis?
2 Why have the OTC treatments been unrewarding?
3 How would you manage this case?

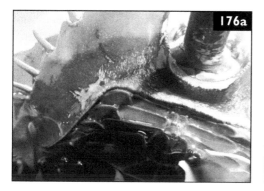

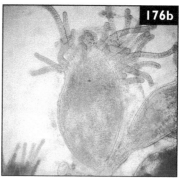

CASE 176 Twelve adult horseshoe crabs (*Limulus polyphemus*), collected from the wild 6 weeks previously, are in quarantine in a 7,500 L (1,980 US gal) system. During their quarantine examinations, three of the animals have white, cotton-like material on the ventral opistosoma (**176a**). Scrape biopsies are examined under direct microscopy (magnification 40×) and show multiple stalked structures; the ends of these structures have bulbs with florets that extend periodically (**176b**).

1 Describe the taxonomy of the horseshoe crab.
2 What type of organism is shown on the images?
3 What treatments might help reduce or eliminate this infection?

CASE 177 As the laboratory veterinarian for a small liberal arts college you are asked by a researcher for assistance in collecting hemolymph from green sea urchins (*Strongylocentrotus droebachiensis*) for a study. It is important that the animals survive this and monthly hemolymph collections for 1 year. Each animal has been marked with a small amount of finger nail polish on a few spines (**177a**, circled). The urchins weigh about 100 g each.

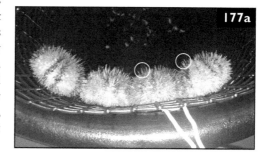

1 What materials will you need?
2 Where will you advise the researcher to place the syringe and needle?
3 Can you estimate how much hemolymph you can take at each sampling time point?

CASE 178 You are presented with acute deaths of koi (*Cyprinus carpio*) in a private pond. The owner, a nurse, examined a few of the dead fish and noted the gills were mottled red/white and the eyes were sunken. The population of approximately 20 mature koi has no prior history of disease problems. It is early May in North Carolina, USA, the water temperature is about 20°C (68°F), and all water parameters are normal according to the owner. While taking the history the owner mentions the fact that he added two new koi to the pond a week ago. The fish were not quarantined and had been purchased from a wholesale facility in California.

1 What infectious disease is at the top of your differential list?
2 How would you confirm your suspicions?
3 What advice would you have for your client with regard to repopulating the pond?

CASE 179

1 What is a fluidized sand filter and how does it function?

CASE 180

1 What is a mangrove filter, how does it work, and what are the advantages and disadvantages?

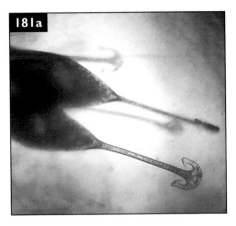

CASE 181 An enthusiastic aquarist finds and shows you a structure she found while examining some aquarium debris under the compound microscope (**181a**). She comments that there were many more of them and sometimes they occurred in clumps.

1 What are these strutures?
2 What are the clinical implications?
3 How would you manage this situation?

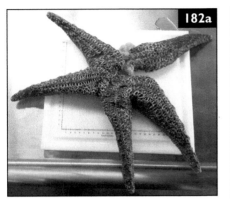

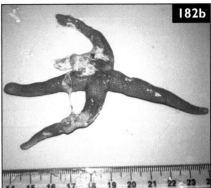

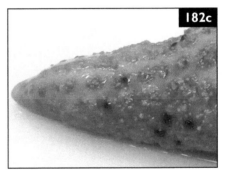

CASE 182 An aquarist/biologist at your facility reports that several dozen sea stars appear bloated and pale. She also reports there are small white lesions on three of the stars at the arm/disc interface. The aquarium recently acquired sea stars from the Washington state coastline.

When you examine the tank, you observe two sea stars with white lesions and two with exposed gonads due to full-thickness ulcerations (*Pisaster ochraceus* and *Henricia* sp., 182a, b respectively). You also notice there are several green urchins (*Strongylocentrotus droebachiensis*) that have dropped spines and have clearly delineated dark patches on their tests. All the sea stars in this tank from the family Asteriidae have common clinical signs including a flattened central disc, swollen rays with poorly adherent tube feet, and white focal lesions on the aboral surface. There are also small (1–2 mm) raised purple spots covering the leather star (*Dermasterias imbricata*) (182c).

1 What is at the top of your differential list and what diagnostic tests would you like to perform?
2 What steps should you take to reduce morbidity and mortality in the echinoderms?

CASE 183

1 What is activated carbon and how does is work?
2 Are there any disadvantages of using activated carbon?

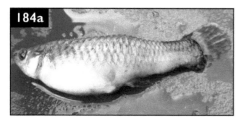

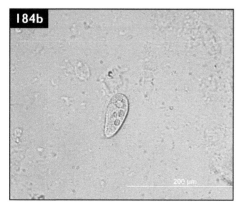

CASE 184 A pet store contacts you because they are experiencing high morbidity and mortality in their heavily stocked fancy guppy (*Poecilia reticulata*) aquaria. Some of the fish have bands of depigmentation along the back in the area of the dorsal fin (**184a**). They have tried a number of over the counter (OTC) antibiotics and parasiticides without success. You test the water and it is within normal limits. Gill biopsies are normal but a biopsy of the depigmented area shows dozens of ciliated protozoans about 50 μm in length (**184b**).

1 What is the most likely diagnosis?
2 Why have the OTC treatments been unrewarding?
3 How would you manage this case?

CASE 185

1 What is zeolite and how does is work?
2 When would the use of zeolite be recommended?

CASE 186

1 How would you recommend treating discharge water from a 1,000 L (264 US gal) hospital tank where fish were treated with an immersion protocol of praziquantel?
2 Would this protocol be acceptable for other types of medications?

CASE 187 There are currently two OIE (World Animal Health Organization) reportable viral diseases of ornamental cyprinids (goldfish and koi).

1 What are these diseases?
2 Discuss their similarities and differences.
3 Where can one find updates and further information about notifiable diseases?

CASE 188 You are called out to see a koi (*Cyprinus carpio*), age and sex unknown, that is floating upside down in a 7,600 L (2,010 US gal) pond following a thunderstorm (188a). The fish occasionally rights itself, but swimming is erratic without effective, purposeful movement from one location to another. Mouth, operculum, and pectoral fin movements are normal, but pelvic, anal, and tail fin movement are decreased or absent. Fins, gills, and skin appear grossly within normal limits.

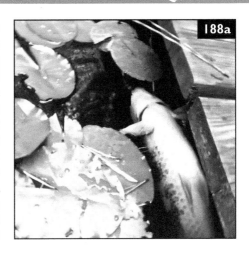

1 What are your differentials?
2 How would you diagnose this case?
3 What are your recommendations to this client?

CASE 189 You have been asked to necropsy two weakfish (*Cynoscion regalis*). The fish were recently caught and there is evidence of trauma on the skin over the dorsal skull on one fish.

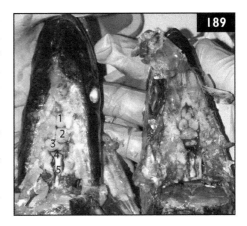

1 Comment on the difference between the two brains in **189**.
2 Identify the anatomic features of the brain that are numbered.
3 What anterior lobe of the brain is not clearly evident or labeled?

CASE 190

1 What is a sand filter and how does it function?

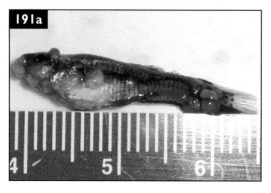

CASE 191 You are presented with a group of pond-reared guppies (*Poecilia reticulata*) (**191a**) that the farmer complains have 'grubs.'

1 What are these 'grubs'?
2 How can you confirm the diagnosis?
3 What is the risk to the fish?
4 How would you manage the problem?

CASE 192 A client calls your office because her recently purchased powder blue tang (*Acanthurus leucosternon*) has a number of discrete and coalescing areas of depigmentation along both flanks above the lateral line (**192a**). The client has tried a number of over the counter (OTC) antibiotics and parasiticides without success. You test the water and it is within normal limits. Gill biopsies are normal but a biopsy of the depigmented area shows dozens of ciliated protozoans about 50 μm in length (**192b**).

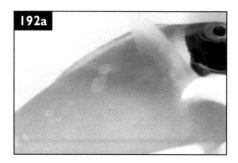
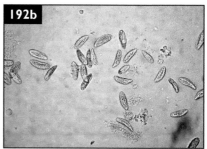

1 What is the most likely diagnosis?
2 Why have the OTC treatments been unrewarding?
3 How would you manage this case?

CASE 193

1 What is ozone filtration and how does it work?
2 What are some disadvantages and limitations of this technology?

CASE 194 A local science museum has just imported a group of marine invertebrates for an exhibit. The shipment included 12 hermit crabs (*Calcinus* sp.), five purple sea urchins (*Arbacia punctulata*), and two orange-ridged sea stars (*Echinaster spinulosus*). All of the animals were placed in the same quarantine tank. Within 24 hours the urchins had died and one of the sea stars was affected by ulcerative dermatitis and 'disintegration syndrome' of two arms (**194a**).

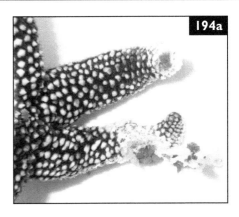

1 How would you manage this case?
2 What changes would you recommend in the future during new animal accession?

CASE 195 You are presented with a mature female apple snail (*Pomacea bridgsii*) that crawled out of its community aquarium and fell to the floor, fracturing its shell. Two significant lesions were noted on the body whirl: a depression fracture and a full-thickness 'U-shaped' crack about 3 cm long (**195a**). The shell tissue surrounding these fractures was unstable.

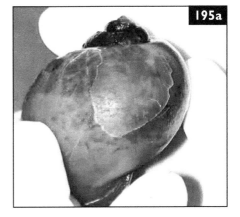

1 Describe gastropod shell anatomy.
2 How would you manage this problem?

CASE 196

1 Discuss the process of making seawater (from a commercial product).
2 What are the advantages and disadvantages compared with natural seawater?

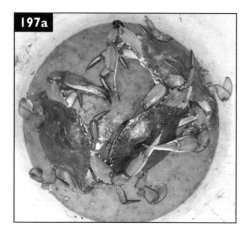

197a

CASE 197 A graduate student in the biology department at the university where you are the consulting laboratory animal veterinarian would like to anesthetize some blue crabs (*Callinectes sapidus*) (197a). You have access to many anesthetic agents used for dogs and cats. You do a literature search and find that a neuroactive steroid anesthetic, recently approved for use in the US, is suitable for blue crab anesthesia.

1 What is this agent?
2 What route and dose would you use for sedation and anesthesia, respectively?
3 What organs are in close proximity to the heart and can be avoided if the syringe and needle are placed appropriately in the center of the arthrodial membrane?

CASE 198 Juvenile yellow stage American eels (*Anguilla rostrata*) in a research colony were radiographed in lateral recumbency to determine the final positions of passive integrated transponder (PIT) tags implanted into the coelomic cavity (198a).

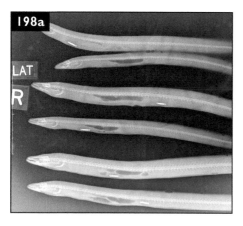

198a

LAT

R

1 What radiographic abnormality is detected incidental to the PIT tag position determination?
2 What is the probable cause of the abnormality?
3 What continent is the source of the responsible agent, and what impacts can it have?

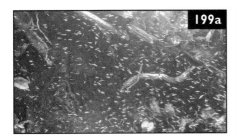
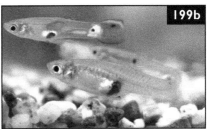

CASE 199 Pictured are two common freshwater aquarium fish, the cardinal tetra (*Paracheirodon axelrodi*; **199a**), and the fancy guppy (*Poeceilia reticulata*; **199b**).

1 Discuss the different reproductive strategies, including basic anatomy and taxonomy, of these small but popular species.

CASE 200 You are presented with a 6-year-old female koi (*Cyprinus carpio*) found acutely down, on the bottom of the pond, on its side (**200a**). Respiratory and pectoral fin movements are normal, but pelvic, anal, and tail fin movement are absent. If the fish is righted by hand, it immediately rolls sideways. There are no external lesions; the fish appears grossly normal.

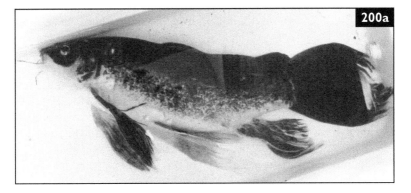

1 What are your differential diagnoses?
2 What additional history would be helpful?
3 What diagnostic tests are needed?
4 What are your recommendations to the client?

CASE 201 An owner presents with an approximately 18-year-old silver dollar fish (*Metynnis* sp.) with a history of tachypnea and anorexia starting 4 days prior. The fish is part of a closed community tank. The last new fish introduced

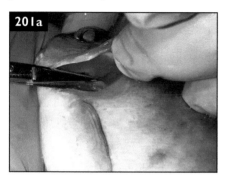

(from a quarantine situation) was over a year ago. There has been no change in diet or husbandry. A water change was performed 3 days prior and it did not improve the fish's clinical signs. The external examination was unremarkable. The fish was in good body condition and weighed 82.8 g. The gill movements were 80 breaths per minute. The gills were observed as being very pale (**201a**).

1 What diagnostic tests would you recommend to the owner?
2 What rule outs would you expect for this fish?
3 How would you manage this case?

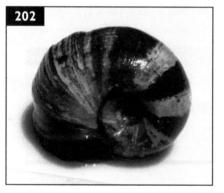

CASE 202 The university where you are employed maintains one of only two known colonies of the extremely rare magnificent ramshorn snail (*Planorbella magnifica*). This freshwater pulmonate belongs to the family Planorbidae.

1 Based on the figure (**202**), is this animal a male or female?
2 What is unusual about many freshwater snails compared with marine snails with regard to respiration?
3 What is unusual about the hemolymph of this family compared with most other invertebrates?

CASE 203

1 What is foam fractionation as it pertains to water quality and life support systems?
2 What is the common name for filtration units that employ this process and give an example of a system where such a unit has utility.

CASE 204 You are the consulting veterinarian for a large outdoor supplies company's expansive indoor life support system. The 400,000 L (105,670 US gal) exhibit houses an array of temperate North American fish including members of the Cyprinidiae, Ictaluridae, and Centrarchidae. The aquarium manager contacts you because a customer pointed out something unusual with one of the catfish (**204**). The fish, along with the rest of the exhibit, have been acting and feeding normally of late. As it turns out the catfish in question does not appear on the census and the aquarist cannot confirm how long the fish has been in the exhibit. It is possible the fish was inappropriately introduced into the exhibit by a customer (an unacceptable but not uncommon practice).

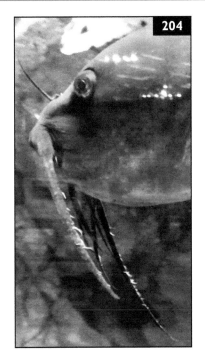

1 What is your top differential based on the clinical presentation and history?
2 Can you describe the life cycle and impact of this organism on fish?
3 How would you manage this situation?

CASE 205 A newly acquired group of pompano (*Trachinotus carolinus*) have been in quarantine for 2 days when the aquarist notices something odd on several of the fish (**205**). As the aquarium's veterinarian, you are asked to identify these organisms and advise the aquarist on a management strategy. Fortunately the fish have been isolated and not exposed to other fish.

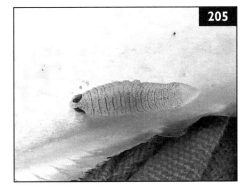

1 What is this organism?
2 How would you manage this problem?

87

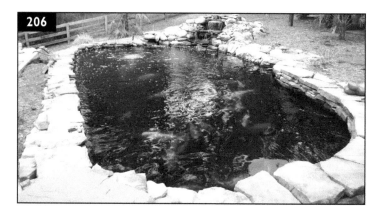

CASE 206 A new client calls your practice about setting up a wellness examination visit for their koi (*Cyprinus carpio*) pond. The pond was part of the real estate deal and the dozen or so mature koi were included (**206**). The new owners have never been fish hobbyists but are interested in learning. They have a number of domestic mammalian pets and are accustomed to veterinary visits and preventive medicine. As far as they know a veterinarian has never visited or worked with the pond or its inhabitants. You would like to determine the volume of the pond and the owners have some information that would be helpful.

1 What measurements would you want to have and how would you calculate volume with these values?
2 Can you name an alternate method that would not require any pond dimension values?

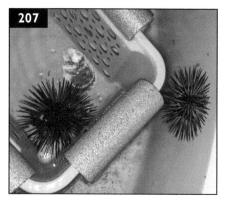

CASE 207 A researcher at the small liberal arts college where you act as the consulting laboratory animal veterinarian would like to anesthetize some purple sea urchins (*Arbacia punctulata*) (**207**). You are experienced with fish but not invertebrates.

1 What commonly used fish anesthetic can be used to anesthetize sea urchins and at what concentration?

CASE 208 You are called out to a 15,200 L (4,010 US gallon) pond that is rapidly losing koi (*Cyprinus carpio*). The pond is located at the front entrance of a business, and the building was pressure washed immediately before fish began showing clinical signs. Now, all of the fish in the pond are either sitting on the bottom, laying over, or dead (**208a**).

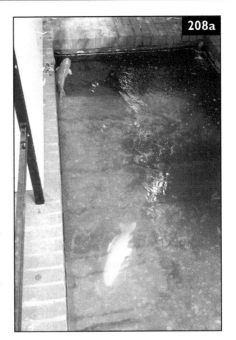

1 What is the likely source of the problem?
2 What steps would you take to help these fish?
3 What is the prognosis?
4 How would you prevent this from happening in the future?

CASE 209 In April you are called to investigate a 11,400 L (3,010 US gal) backyard pond containing various koi and goldfish. Several koi have died

over the past week, and most of the remaining koi have stopped eating and are acting lethargic. You observe a few koi swimming with their head down. Affected koi have sunken eyes and a notched nose (**209**, arrows). The goldfish are not affected. The pond was established 5 years ago, has excellent filtration, and water quality appears normal. A month earlier, the client had introduced a couple of new koi, and those fish are also affected.

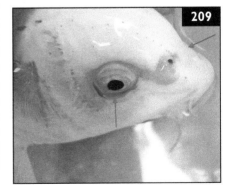

1 What is your primary differential?
2 How would you confirm your suspicion?
3 What can you do to help the remaining fish?
4 How can the client reduce the chance of a similar event happening again?

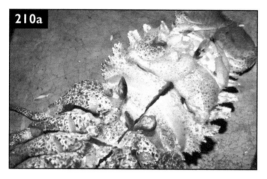

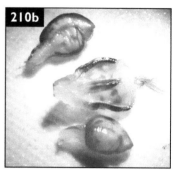

CASE 210 The aquarium you consult for is preparing to open a Pacific tropical mixed-species crustacean exhibit. They have a source for slipper lobsters (*Scyllarides astori*), but it is a live seafood company, and in a roundabout way you obtained an image of one of their lobsters ready for the grill (**210a**) at a local restaurant. You are friendly with the chef and she knows your interest in odd things found on and in her whole seafood items. She cooked the lobster but not before removing the strange organisms for your inspection (**210b**).

1　What are these organisms?
2　How would you manage this issue?

CASE 211 The invertebrate curator of the large aquarium where you work is concerned about some of her moon jellies (*Aurelia aurita*). She notes that about

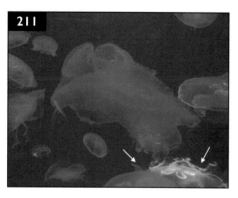

10% of them seem to be inside out, are unable to feed, and appear to be shrinking. You inspect the tank and observe that approximately one in 10 jellies are unable to move normally and the bell is curled opposite to the normal conformation (**211**, arrows).

1　What is this syndrome called?
2　What is known about it?
3　How would you manage the problem?

CASE 212 Pictured is an image of a blood film from a goldfish (*Carassius auratus*) (**212**).

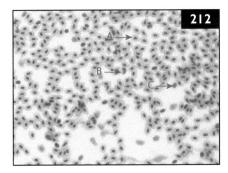

1 Name the cells indicated by the letters and arrows.

CASE 213 One of the aquarists where you work asks to have a cuttlefish (*Sepia* sp.) with a dorsal mantle lesion examined. Based on your through-the-tank examination you decide a closer look and possible biopsy are warranted.

1 How would you anesthetize the cuttlefish for this procedure? Please include details on induction, maintenance, and recovery.

CASE 214 You are the veterinarian of record for a small university Institutional Animal Care and Use Committee (IACUC) and a question arises about the maximum volume of blood collected from each individual in a population of goldfish (*Carassius auratus*). The researcher (very new to fish research) only needs a single blood sample from each fish but would like to obtain as much as possible for current and future studies.

1 What information would you like to have before commenting?
2 Based on this information how would you calculate an estimate for safe blood collection volume?
3 What anatomic site would you recommend the IACUC approved researchers use for the blood samples?

CASE 215 A pet fish owner is moving from California to North Carolina. They own six fresh water fish and are interested in moving them too. Two of the fish are at least 15 years old and range in size from 2 to 16 cm in length. It would take approximately 45 hours to drive the fish across the country.

1 What recommendations would you have for the owner regarding safe and efficient transportation?
2 How would you package the fish for transport?

CASE 216 A young tenure track professor in the biology department of the university you serve as the laboratory animal veterinarian is interested in collecting hemolymph from bivalve mollusks for an important research study. She wants to collect samples once a month for a year, therefore survival of the animals is critical to her work.

1 How can this be accomplished?

CASE 217 A client with a well established koi (*Cyprinus carpio*) pond has lost several koi over the past week. The remaining fish have stopped eating and are clustered together at the bottom of the pond. There have been no new fish added to the pond for several years. The client does not routinely perform partial water changes, and only 'tops off' the pond with dechlorinated city water as needed. There have been extremely heavy rains for the past month. Water testing reveals the following: pH ≤6.0 (below range of test kit, **217**); ammonia ≥4 ppm (above range of test kit); total alkalinity (kH) = 0 ppm; nitrite 0; nitrate >200 ppm (above range of test kit).

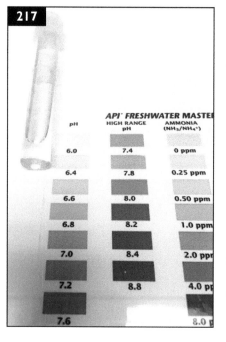

1 What is your primary differential for this situation?
2 Explain the water test results for your client.
3 What steps would you take to resolve this problem, and what special precautions should you take?

CASE 218

1 What is a canister filter and how does it function?

CASE 219 It is early one Monday morning and you receive a call from the head curator of a large marine temperate exhibit. She is clearly distressed, with urgency in her voice. While doing her rounds before getting to her office space she noticed a hose laying across the floor and leading into the trench drain that returned water to the filter system. Since she was the first person in, the hose had to have been running all night. That is at least 15 hours of fresh water (FW) spilling into a salt water (SW) aquarium system.

1 A number of actions are required. List them in order of priority.
2 What precautions could be taken to prevent this from happening in the future?
3 What is a beneficial side effect of lowered salinity?

CASE 220 A large research colony of green research sea urchins (*Strongylocentrotus droebachiensis*) (**220**) is experiencing high morbidity and mortality linked to a gram-negative bacterium sensitive to enrofloxacin.

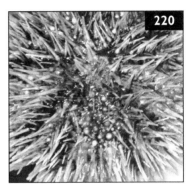

1 What intracoelomic (ICe) dosing regimen would you recommend?
2 What immersion dosing regimen would be appropriate?

CASE 221 You are pulling weekend duty at the natural science museum where you are employed as the veterinarian. Your pager goes off and you are summoned to the program animal holding area by the Sunday volunteer, who is very concerned that one of the California sea hares (*Aplysia californica*) is bleeding to death, and the water is becoming red with its blood.

1 Briefly describe a sea hare.
2 On your way to address the issue you stop and patiently answer a visitor's questions about one of the exhibits. Why are you not in a rush to save the hemorrhaging sea hare?
3 If the sea hare was truly 'bleeding' (losing hemolymph), what color would it be and why?
4 If you had to anesthetize a sea hare, what chemical and concentration would be appropriate?

CASE 1

1 What is your next diagnostic step considering the delicate nature of bonnethead sharks? Testing stray electrical current and copper are always warranted in cephalofoil sharks. Both of these were tested and considered normal before proceeding. A full examination requiring capture of an adult can be stressful but may be necessary. An iSTAT or similar device is recommended to monitor blood pH and lactic acid during shark examinations. In this case, a quick examination of the gill slits found numerous monogeneans that were confirmed with microscopic examination as *Erpocotyle tiburonis* (1). The previous praziquantel immersions should have resolved this condition.

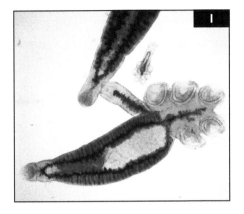

2 Had there been evidence of lactic acidosis how would you manage this problem? Sodium bicarbonate can be given in the dorsal fin sinus, ventral tail vein, or IM at 1.0 mEq/kg as often as necessary. Juvenile bonnethead sharks are easy to catch at the surface, although their small size can make administration of bicarbonate difficult. Using oxygen to saturate the water to 115–150% can alleviate lactic acidosis, and staff agreed to a quick examination on a bonnethead juvenile despite no findings on necropsy.

CASE 2

1 Why are there still monogeneans present in Case 1 despite the praziquantel treatment and how will you proceed using the same drug? Repeat use of certain chemotherapeutics can alter the biological filter, which adapts to use certain drugs as carbon sources. Without complete disinfection between quarantines, the biofilter became accustomed to consuming praziquantel, which allowed a monogenean infection to occur. Juveniles were first affected due to their small size and naivety. In this case, a 3.0 ppm dose was administered with water samples collected for validation by high pressure liquid chromatography. Praziquantel levels were found to fall below therapeutic levels within 3 hours instead of the usual 7–10 days. The infection was controlled by several methods including one 10.0 ppm praziquantel 4 hour bath, two 10.0 ppm chloroquine prolonged immersions, and a slow reduction in salinity to 20 ppt to reduce monogenean egg fecundity. This case also highlights the need to have an experienced veterinarian on staff for examinations and necropsy to assist aquarists with disease detection.

2 What is the correlation between tank temperature and pathogen-induced dermatitis in the bonnethead sharks (*Sphyrna tiburo*) in Case 1? Four common pathogens in captive bonnethead sharks are *Fusarium solani*, *Amyloodinium*, monogeneans, and parasitic copepods. The latter three organisms are obligate

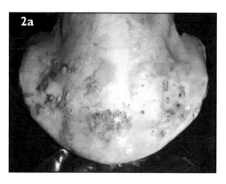

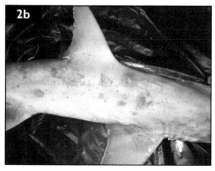

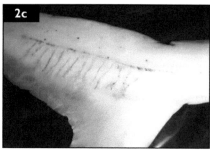

pathogens that are amenable to treatment. *F. solani* is an opportunistic pathogen and ubiquitous fungus in salt water. Immunocompromized sharks can succumb to a chronic *F. solani* dermatitis that is very difficult to treat. Small abrasions, overcrowding, pregnancy, poor water quality, or other infection may predispose a bonnethead shark to the fungal infection, which initially presents as ulcers along the head and lateral line system (**2a–c**). Raising the tank water temperature to 26.7–27.8°C (80–82°F) or more appears effective in combination with good filtration (ozone, UV light) to prevent or reduce incidence of *F. solani* infections.

CASE 3

1 What are your top differentials for the acute mortality? It is possible the traumatic lesions were more extensive than initially determined and caused death due to organ failure. Also, since the hospital tank was empty, a large fish may have caused a rapid change in the water quality, such as decreased DO level or increased ammonia levels, if the tank was not properly cycled.

2 What further testing do you want to do? Water quality testing and radiography.

3 **What abnormalities would you expect to find?** Radiographs confirm there are no fractures and no deeper lesions or internal contusions are noted on necropsy. However, the gills are dark red to purple, confirming the suspicion of ammonia toxicity. Water quality testing reveals the ammonia is 1.5 ppm total ammonia nitrogen (TAN) and the pH is 8.5. All other results are within normal limits, including DO.

4 **How would you manage the problem identified by your diagnostic work up?** Treatments for ammonia toxicity include an immediate water change and the addition of biofiltration from an established tank or the addition of 'seeding' products that contain nitrifying microorganisms that convert ammonia to nitrite. An easily overlooked aspect of ammonia toxicity is its increased harmful nature with increased pH. Unionized ammonia (NH_3) is more toxic than ionized ammonia or ammonium (NH_4^+). Thus a lower level of TAN is more likely to be lethal at a pH of 8.5 than a pH of 7.0. The DO level should be increased to 110–120% to increase the concentration gradient across the gills and ease oxygen consumption by the fish until the gills have healed. Frequent water quality testing and water changes should be conducted until the life support system is established and the ammonia normalizes.

CASE 4

1 **How is the clinical presentation of goiter usually different in elasmobranchs as compared with bony fish?** In sharks and rays the swelling is usually in the ventral gular area and not directly associated with the gills (4).

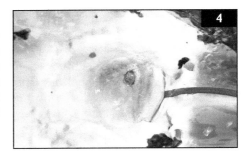

CASE 5

1 **What is your top differential diagnosis?** Thyroid hyperplasia (goiter) should be your top differential based on the appearance and location of the mass/swelling. The goiter may be unilateral or bilateral. Goiter has been identified in many species of both freshwater and saltwater fish. Goiter in fish is a result of iodide (I^-) deficiency, which is the form of iodine available for uptake by the thyroid gland. Deficiency may be a result of water depleted of iodide, dietary deficiency of iodide, or by goiterogenic compounds. In bony fish, other tumors of the oral cavity and pharyngeal structures do occur but are less common. In elasmobranchs, trauma or local infection are other possible causes for the swelling but are less common. Aspiration or biopsy can be used to confirm a diagnosis but is usually reserved until

Answers

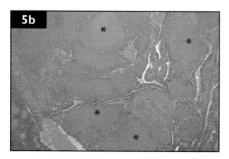

there is no improvement with treatment. Aspiration and cytology typically reveal blood cells but can sometimes yield viscous clear to yellow colloid. Biopsy is usually diagnostic and can help distinguish between hyperplasia and neoplasia. Numerous colloid filled nodules were present (**5b**, asterisks) consistent with thyroid hyperplasia.

2 What are your recommendations for treatment and prevention of this problem?
The most common treatment for goiter is oral supplementation with iodide, typically in the form of potassium iodide (KI) salt at a dose of 10 mg/kg body weight once weekly. Alternatively, water supplementation with KI salt or Lugol's iodine at or above the amount found in natural seawater may be effective, but caution must be used as elemental iodine in Lugol's can be toxic if overdosed. Treatment may need to be continued for several months or longer to see significant reduction in the size of the goiter. Oral supplemental treatment with thyroxine at 0.02 mg/kg may be of benefit in treating any concurrent hypothyroidism, and decrease the over production of thyrotropin-releasing hormone and thyroid-stimulating hormone, but it is not typically required. Some residual hypertrophied tissue may remain despite resolution of the clinical disease. Measures should be initiated to prevent recurrence and new cases.

Prevention of goiter should focus on maintenance of sufficient iodide levels in the water and/or oral supplementation in the diet and correction of elevated nitrate (NO_3^-) levels. The preventive method used must be tailored to the fish species and system being evaluated. Iodide levels in natural seawater are in the range 0.01–0.06 mg/L, but they can vary widely and be much lower in freshwater. Recommended tank iodide levels to prevent goiter in marine tanks are 0.10–0.15 µM (0.02–0.03 mg/L). Testing for iodide rather than iodate (IO_3) is recommended but requires special methodologies that can be challenging.

Biological utilization and oxidation of iodide are the main ways it is depleted in aquaria. Replenishment is most often accomplished through regular water changes or commercially available liquid supplements added weekly. Ozonation of seawater for disinfection rapidly oxidizes iodide to iodate, resulting in an iodide depleted environment despite water changes or supplementation. In this situation, dietary supplementation may be a more effective therapy than water supplementation.

Most natural seafood items and commercially prepared fish foods contain sufficient iodine to prevent goiter but natural freshwater items such as fish or shrimp can be deficient. Some raw terrestrial plants (broccoli, kale, cabbage) also contain goiterogens and should not be fed in excess. Minimum dietary requirements for iodide are not available for most fish species, but 2.8 mg iodide/kg of food (0.00028%) is one recommendation for freshwater fish. Iodide has been safely supplemented to large marine fish, sharks, and rays in a commercial multivitamin (Mazuri® Shark and Ray tabs) at a rate of 1,000 mg/kg of food (0.1%) and in gel food (Mazuri® Omnivore gel diet) at 20 mg/kg of food (0.002%) for smaller fish. Potassium iodide salt 20–1,000 mg/kg of food can also be used to coat natural food items or be added to gel diets if commercial products are not available or additional supplementation is indicated.

In systems with high levels of nitrate, naturally occurring water levels and dietary content of iodide may not be sufficient to prevent goiter. Nitrate is considered to be goiterogenic by competitively inhibiting the uptake of iodide by the thyroid gland. Recent studies have shown that previously recommended upper limit nitrate levels of 70 mg/L (NO_3-N) can induce thyroid hyperplasia in sharks despite having normal water iodide concentrations. Increased dietary supplementation may be beneficial in situations where low nitrate levels are unable to be maintained.

CASE 6

1 Can you identify the pathologic lesion? There is a mesenteric torsion of the mid-intestinal tract. The affected intestine and mesentery are severely congested and showing signs of necrosis.

Further examination revealed a stomach full of large pieces of broccoli stem (**6b**) and a distal intestine full of fine plant material. No other abnormalities were identified on gross examination or histopathology. The final diagnosis was intestinal torsion, intestinal necrosis, and cardiovascular shock. It is suspected that the large amount of ingested broccoli played a role in this unusual case. Excess fiber ingestion has not previously been reported as a problem in marine angelfish.

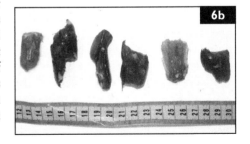

CASE 7

1 What questions do you want to ask the aquarist? Is this the only animal affected? Have there been any new additions to the exhibit recently? Have there been any recent mortalities? Have there been any changes in the life support system?

You learn from the aquarists that no new fish have been added, but 15 of the 20 seahorses in the exhibit are showing similar signs with swellings along the

Answers

body, and some have exophthalmos. The exhibit's spotfin butterflyfish has similar lesions, especially in the fins. All are alive but many are in poor condition.

2 What diagnostic tests do you want to perform? Gill and skin biopsies of the butterflyfish and fine needle aspiration of at least one sea horse dermal swelling. The swellings of the seahorse are easily reduced when gas is removed via aspiration (**7a, b** show two seahorses with gas bubbles on the snouts). Gas emboli are observed on a wet mount of a gill clip from the spotfin butterflyfish.

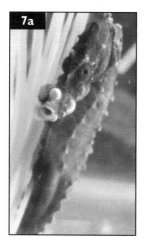 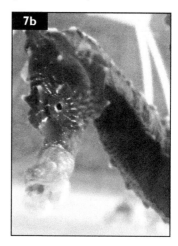

3 Based on your findings what is the most likely diagnosis? These results are diagnostic for gas bubble disease likely due to supersaturation. Other confirmatory diagnostics include a visual of microbubbles throughout the tank, or testing the DO level and total gas pressure (using a tensiometer). A close examination of the life support system shows a pinpoint hole in one of the lines from the pump to the aquarium. This pinpoint puncture is allowing room air to be added to the water going directly to the exhibit. The hose is quickly replaced. All animals are treated with a dose of the carbonic anhydrase inhibitor acetazolamide at 2.5 mg/kg IM. The animals in the worst condition are placed in a recompression chamber to a maximum pressure of 2 atmosphere and slowly decompressed over several hours. All animals recover within 24 hours.

CASE 8

1 What diagnostics do you want to conduct? Moderate buphthalmos is observed with diffuse corneal edema, an area of loose corneal tissue, and multiple gas bubbles within the anterior chamber. Fluorescein stain uptake occurred on a 2 × 1 cm zone of the superior cornea (**8a**) and indicates a corneal ulceration.

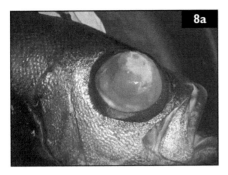
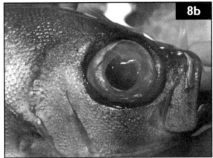

2 What procedures and/or treatments would you perform? In this case, after applying topical antibiotics, an aspiration of the anterior chamber produced 2 ml of gas, causing the globe to return to normal conformation with a slightly concave cornea (**8b**). Loose corneal tissue was gently removed from the ulcerated region using a cotton-tipped applicator, and a grid keratotomy was performed. Further treatment included broad-spectrum systemic and topical antibiotics q 3 days, meloxicam 0.3 mg/kg IM q 3 days, acetazolamide 2.5 mg/kg IM q 1 week, and TruSopt® (dorzolamide hydrochloride) ophthalmic solution 1–2 drops topically q 3 days when handled for other treatments. Frequency of topical medications can be increased based on the demeanor of the species and ability to withstand daily handling.

CASE 9

1 What is the most likely diagnosis? The degenerative condition known as head and lateral line erosion (HLLE).

2 What questions would you like to ask the owner? How long have the lesions been present? Can you describe the tank set up, water quality, and what you are feeding the fish? Have you recently used carbon as part of the filtration?

3 Describe HLLE for your client and provide information regarding prevention and treatment options. HLLE is a disfiguring but rarely fatal degenerative condition of marine fish. Similar lesions occur in freshwater fish, often referred to as hole in the head disease, but have a different etiology. The exact pathogenesis of this syndrome is unclear; there are multiple causative scenarios reported that may result in this condition. Improper nutrition, inadequate lighting, stray voltage, copper treatment, water quality, and carbon filtration have all been implicated.

The most common and only reproducible cause is the use of carbon filtration for periods of 2 weeks or longer. Some reports suggest that carbon particles directly result in the lesions through mechanical contact with the fish's skin and lateral line cells. Others suggest that prolonged carbon filtration removes organic components from the water resulting in the condition. In either case, limiting the use and duration of carbon filtration, and providing near 100% water replenishment after carbon filtration, are very important to preventing HLLE.

Surgeonfish, tangs, and butterfly fish are particularly prone to developing this condition. Avoidance of these fish species would be recommended in situations where the etiology has not been identified.

If HLLE is identified early, within several weeks of onset, and the cause identified and corrected, there is a good chance for partial to full reversal. With small lesions (<5 mm) that are older and static, light débridement under sedation using a scalpel blade similar to a skin scrape once a week for 3–4 weeks may be sufficient to stimulate skin regeneration. Caution must be used not to create traumatic wounds during débridement. Long-term (months to years) and larger lesions will not heal without medical treatment. Lesions are rarely progressive once the etiology is removed.

Regranex® (becaplermin 0.01%) is a commercial product available for medical treatment of HLLE. It is a gel containing recombinant platelet derived growth factor approved for topical use in wound healing for humans. Application of the gel to the lesions for a period of 10 seconds after light débridement once weekly is

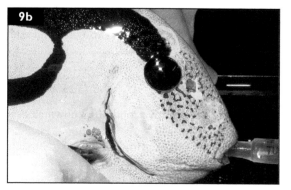

recommended. The length of treatment can range from 3 weeks to many months depending on the duration and severity of the lesions. Results are generally quite good (9b); however, high cost and relatively short expiration periods may limit the availability and practicality of this treatment.

CASE 10

1 Is skin scraping these lesions appropriate? Yes.

2 What is the top differential for these clinical signs and should the whole school of fish be culled and another batch obtained? A diagnosis of lymphocystis was made. Lymphocystis disease, a chronic self-limiting disease of both marine and freshwater fishes, is caused by an iridovirus. It rarely becomes systemic and generally affects dermal fibroblasts, causing them to hypertrophy. Its cause is considered multifactorial but has been known to be brought on by stress and is commonly seen after transportation of teleosts. There is no known treatment. In this instance, stress among the fish was reduced with the addition of more structures to provide hide spots, and more frequent feedings. The lesions resolved after several weeks without any complications.

CASE 11

1 Should the other exhibits in this system be suspected of having a monogenean infestation? Yes, ectoparasites are known to pass easily through filtration systems into other exhibits. Also, in general, the same aquarist will service all the exhibits in their section, potentially spreading the ectoparasites directly to each exhibit if proper biosecurity measures are not practiced.

2 Would copper sulfate, a common drug used for treatment of ectoparasites, be indicated for use throughout the entire 82,800 L (21,875 US gal) system? No, copper sulfate would be contraindicated in this particular situation. Copper sulfate is not tolerated well by elasmobranchs and is lethal to invertebrates.

3 Devise a treatment plan for treating the entire system. In this instance the entire system was treated with long-term praziquantel immersions at 2.5 mg/L q 3 days for a total of three treatments. After administration of the praziquantel during the evening hours all filtration units were turned off for the duration of the treatment. At the end of the treatment period, a large water change and backwash was performed and then the treatment regimen repeated. After the praziquantel treatment concluded, the exhibit where the mongeneans was initially found was isolated. All invertebrates were removed from this exhibit, leaving only teleosts, and the exhibit underwent a 1 hour formalin immersion at 150 mg/L q 7 days for three treatments. Extra airstones were supplied to the exhibit during the formalin treatment to combat the drug's oxygen depriving effects. Once the formalin treatment concluded a 50% water change was performed. Invertebrates were given a 1 minute freshwater bath before being placed back into the exhibit to prevent reseeding the system with any *Neobenedenia* that may have hitchhiked onto the invertebrates. Approximately 2 weeks after all treatments were completed, multiple animals throughout the many exhibits were captured and skin scrapes and gill clips were performed. No ectoparasites were noted on any animal. The gallery was considered clear of the monogenean infestation.

4 How much praziquantel would be needed for one treatment in the 82,800 L (21,875 US gal) system at a dosage of 2.5 mg/L? 207 grams.

CASE 12

1 Describe the lesions seen in 12a, b. Image **12a** reveals multiple raised cream-colored to gray irregular nodular cutaneous masses. Image **12b** is an unstained wet mount at low magnification (10× objective) revealing a large cystic mass with a distinct cell wall. There is no apparent nucleus within the structure. The gross lesions and wet mount images represent either lymphocystis or epitheliocystis.

2 What are the two most likely causes for the lesions seen in the porkfish? Epitheliocystis is caused by intracellular, gram-negative bacteria in the Order Chlamydiales. There is a high diversity and host specificity associated with this pathogen; therefore, this disease can be highly pathogenic and cause severe mortalities, especially in juvenile fish. Although the organism is considered to be distinct and separate from those of the Chlamydiaceae, tetracycline is considered to be a treatment option to reduce mortality. A presumptive diagnosis of epitheliocystis was made in this case based on the gross lesions, wet mount findings, high morbidity and mortality, and rapid response to tetracycline treatment. However, the pathology report of one of the deceased fish indicated lymphocystis based on histopathology findings. Lymphocystis is caused by an iridovirus (Iridoviridae) and is considered to be less pathogenic than related viruses such as ranaviruses and megalocytiviruses. Lymphocystis is not typically associated with high mortalities. The gross lesions of lymphocystis and epitheliocystis can appear similar. Lymphocystis lesions develop over the course of days and can last for weeks. Lymphocystis lesions are caused by clusters of enlarged fibroblasts (over 50,000 times the size of a normal fibroblast) and most affected fish recover without treatment after a few weeks. This case demonstrates a disconnection between the pathologic findings and the clinical course of the disease. It is possible that this case represents a rare form of lymphocystis infection and the apparent response to the tetracycline therapy was mere coincidence.

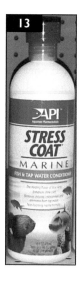

CASE 13

1 Why are the fish developing these symptoms and what should be done to treat this problem and safely move forward with acclimation? These fish are exhibiting symptoms of ammonia toxicity and probable subclinical acidosis. Ammonia (NH_3) at low pH is converted to ammonium (NH_4^+), which is significantly less toxic to fish, so the low pH in the shipping water was protecting the fish from ammonia toxicity. As the pH of the acclimation water is increasing from the addition of buffered seawater and the removal of built-up CO_2 by aeration, NH_3 is rising and toxicity signs developing. Immediate steps to remove or neutralize the ammonia must be taken. This is most easily done by the addition of one of the many commercial products that rapidly bind ammonia (**13**). It can also be accomplished by using seawater with a chemically lowered pH to dilute or flush out the ammonia while in its less toxic form. Temperature stress and pH stress should be avoided by continuing a slow acclimation and regular monitoring. A good general rule of thumb is to increase pH by no more than 0.5 per hour and temperature by 2°C (3.6°F) per hour.

2 How could this problem be prevented with future shipments? This situation can be prevented by discarding the majority of shipping water and adding an ammonia neutralizer/binder prior to starting the acclimation process. In extreme cases of prolonged shipping times (>36 hours) and low pH (<6.0) the receiving system pH may need to be partially lowered and raised slowly over 24 hours or more to allow the fish to metabolically adjust back to their preferred pH range.

CASE 14

1 What are your top differentials? Thyroid hyperplasia, abscess or granuloma, parasitic cyst, and neoplasia.

2 What diagnostics do you want to perform? Fine needle aspirate with cytology, lancing/debriding, and culture and sensitivity.

3 Based on the results of your diagnostic tests what is the condition and how will you proceed? A fine needle aspirate of the mass is unproductive. An attempt to extrude any granulomatous material or parasitic cyst by lancing the ventral aspect of the mass is also unproductive. A culture of the mass is negative for aerobic bacteria and fungus. Based on the location, appearance, and rule out of infection, the mass is most likely a hyperplastic thyroid due to lack of iodine. The majority of iodine uptake for bony fish is from the environment rather than from food. Artificial saltwater or certain sterilization techniques, such as ozonation, can cause a low level of free iodine in the water. Testing environmental iodine can be difficult as other halogens interfere with the results (i.e. bromine and chlorine). Addition of Lugol's 1% iodine to a level of 0.06 ppm, which is the general oceanic iodine level, significantly reduced the mass over 6 weeks to a thickness of 3 mm (**14b**), at which time treatment was discontinued. A histologic section confirmed a hyperplastic thyroid (**14c**).

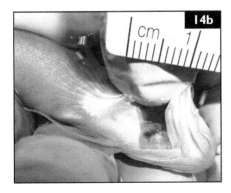
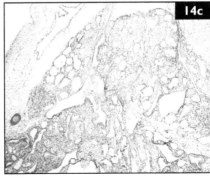

Answers

CASE 15

1 What are the possible causes for this condition? Dysbarism, which includes barotrauma and decompression sickness, is a possible etiology for gas buphthalmia. Gases in enclosed cavities can expand and dissolved gases in the blood can come out of solution during rapid ascension from depth. This condition typically involves swim bladder expansion and gas buphthalmia of both eyes. There is no history of significant depth change in this case.

Gas supersaturation of the tank water is another possible cause for gas buphthalmia. Increased partial pressure of gases, typically nitrogen or oxygen, in the water enter the fish through the gills and come out of solution within various tissues, frequently the gills, subcutaneous spaces, and around the eyes. Supersaturation can occur in water collected at depth (wells), from mechanical addition of gases such as vigorous aeration (waterfalls or pump cavitation), and from biological addition of gasses (e.g. photosynthesis) in ponds. In this case, a saturometer was used to determine that the total gas pressure (%) in the tank was mildly elevated and the likely cause for the gas buphthalmia.

There have been cases of gas buphthalmia that do not involve ascension from depth or gas supersaturation of the water. Infectious causes include bacterial, fungal, or parasitic diseases within or behind the eye, but seem to occur less commonly. Trauma to the eye may also be a cause for gas buphthalmia, although the mechanism is unclear. Typically, such cases are unilateral and would be a good rule out for this case if supersaturation was not detected.

2 What are the treatment options and prognosis for this fish? Mechanical removal of the gas from behind or within the eye can be performed with an appropriately sized syringe using the smallest needle possible to reach the gas pocket (**15b**). Multiple aspirations over the course of treatment may be required if new gas forms. A combination of an antibiotic, anti-inflammatory, and a carbonic anhydrase inhibitor administered by IM injection is the mainstay of medical therapy. Therapy should be continued for several treatments after no new gas is formed in or behind the eye.

Environmental methods such as cooling the water or caging the fish at depth have been suggested as possible treatments to assist in solubilizing and removing the gas. Hyperbaric tank treatment has been used with good success to treat fish with dysbarism collected from depth. Recently this treatment has shown great promise in treating gas buphthalmia in captive fish regardless of the cause. A custom hyperbaric tank (**15c**) can be built at a reasonable cost. Since it is filled with pressurized water instead of oxygen it does not carry the same danger of explosive rupture. Pressure can be adjusted from 0 to 80 psi, the equivalent depth of 0–51.8 m (0–170 ft), and is pressurized until the eye returns to normal or it stops reducing in size. Often the fish will become negatively buoyant because of concurrent compression of the swim bladder. Pressure is maintained for 24 hours

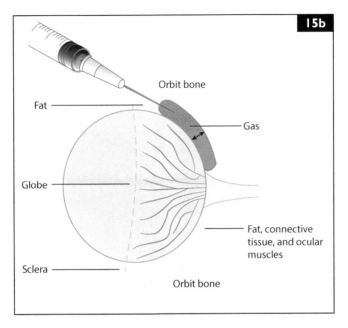

Orbit bone

Fat

Gas

Globe

Fat, connective tissue, and ocular muscles

Sclera

Orbit bone

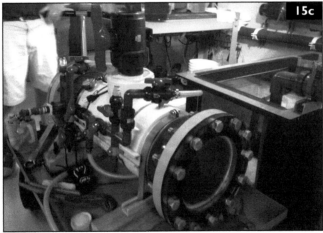

and then slowly reduced by 10 psi every few hours while monitoring the eye for enlargement and the fish for positive buoyancy. If that occurs slower adjustment may be necessary. Medical therapy for any underlying disease process must be addressed and may need to be continued until residual tissue swelling is resolved. The treatment duration is typically much shorter than when aspiration is used to remove the gas.

Prognosis for survival for fish with gas buphthalmia that receive medical treatment is good. Prognosis for vision is good when gas is located only behind the eye but is guarded when gas is visible within the globe because significant mechanical damage to the retina often occurs. Ultrasonographic images show a normal fish eye (15d) and a fish eye with detached retina post-gas buphthalmia treatment (15e). Sequelae to non-treatment may involve rupture of the globe, development of phthisis bulbi, or secondary infection and death.

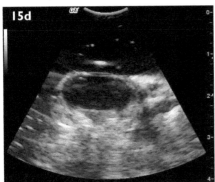 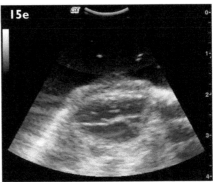

Surgical removal of the eye is an additional option if treatment is impractical or unsuccessful.

CASE 16

1 **What diagnostic tests would you recommend?** Fin biopsy microscopy in addition to standard diagnostics, including gill biopsy and microscopy of an impression smear of scales and mucus or skin scrape, should be considered in all fish quarantine health management plans. These diagnostics will aid in the evaluation of overall health and in screening for the presence of external parasites. In this case, visual in-tank evaluations of fish attitude and behavior revealed no abnormal findings. Physical examinations were performed under general anesthesia and other than the lesions described above, findings were within normal limits. Body condition scores were reported as 2.5 to 3/5, indicating that these fish were well conditioned. Fecal samples collected opportunistically during anesthesia were evaluated and no ova or organisms were observed in the samples. Gills appeared healthy and no abnormal findings were reported from skin scrape microscopy. However, microscopy (~40× magnification) of the fin lesions revealed gross wart-like masses circumscribing the outer edge of the dorsal fin (16c).

2 **Based on your findings what is your top differential diagnosis?** Lymphocystis disease is a self-limiting iridoviral disease caused by *Lymphocystivirus* or *Lymphocystis disease virus* (LCDV), often described in freshwater, estuarine,

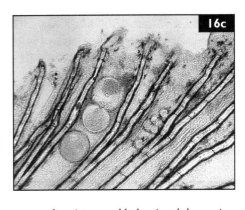

and marine fish species. The disease is named for the hypertrophied viron-filled fibroblastic cells called lymphocycsts that can develop in skin, gill, or fin tissue of infected fish. Detection of lymphocysts via microscopic evaluation of biopsy samples targeting papilloma-like lesions of the fins, gills, or skin is pathognomonic for this disease. This disease is usually associated with shipping stress or environmental stress including changes in temperature, water chemistry, and behavioral dynamics.

3 How would you manage this case? There are no specific treatments or medications targeting lymphocystis disease in fish. Although the papilloma-like lesions are quite disfiguring, they are generally temporary, and resolve spontaneously over several weeks. Unless nodules become mechanically obstructive due to size or location, and need to be surgically removed, fish often continue to feed normally and remain unaffected in attitude and behavior. Supportive care and surgical removal of nodules may be indicated in severe cases. Effort should be made to reduce stress and maintain water quality. A fish quarantine health management plan should be in place with a standard 30–60 day quarantine period for new fish to reduce exposure and spread of the disease.

CASE 17

1 What type of agent is propofol? Propofol is a commonly used anesthetic approved for use in humans, dogs, and cats. It works by enhancing the gamma-aminobutyric acid receptor, resulting in CNS depression and immobility.

2 How can it be applied to fish? Propofol can be administered IV to fish, but is more easily used as an immersion anesthetic (**17**). It can be used for sedation for transport or to produce general anesthesia for examinations or procedures. Typical induction dose is approximately 5 mg/L.

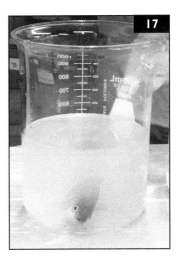

3 Is this compound approved for use in fish intended for human consumption? Propofol is not approved for use in fish and should not be administered to fish in the food chain.

Answers

CASE 18

1 Describe the gross lesions present in 18a. The most obvious lesion presented in this image involves a collection of gas emboli within the anterior chamber of the eye. Secondly, the full outer circumference of the lens can be visualized, indicating an anterior lens luxation.

2 What diagnostic tests would you like to employ other than physical examination? Gill and skin biopsy, fecal collection, fluoroscein corneal staining, aspiration of the affected eye plus sample processing, and examination of the other fish in the aquarium.

3 Based on your diagnostic findings what is your diagnosis? Anterior lens luxation. Moderate to severe ocular trauma is the most likely diagnosis for anterior lens luxation in this case. Intraspecific and interspecific interactions or aggression are common in aquaria, especially during feeding or with reproductive maturation of fish in the system. Trauma can be caused directly from tank-mate interactions or can be self-induced when fish swim at high speeds in relatively confined aquaria. Intraocular gas emboli observed in fish are often an indication of gas bubble disease (GBD) and are related to gas supersaturation within the water of the aquarium. GBD should be considered a reasonable differential in this case. However, the only gas emboli observed were associated with the right eye and lens luxation of a single fish. No other evidence was found in this fish or in several other fish evaluated. While corneal damage was not observed, it is possible that the initial insult involved a corneal perforation. This could explain the occurrence of gas emboli in the single affected eye in the absence of GBD. Other than the eye lesions noted above, physical examination revealed no abnormalities. Body condition score was reported as 2.5/5, indicating that the fish was adequately conditioned. A fecal sample collected opportunistically during anesthesia was evaluated and no ova or organisms were observed. Gills appeared healthy with no signs of intravascular gas emboli and no abnormal findings reported from skin scrape microscopy. Three other fish of the same species and one Florida pompano were also evaluated from the same aquarium system. No abnormalities were noted. There was no growth reported from fungal and bacterial cultures performed on fine needle aspirate fluid collected from the eye.

4 How will you manage the case? Fine needle aspiration of gas and humor with a single intraocular administration of antibiotics (**18c**) was performed

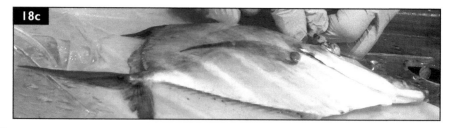

18c

under anesthesia and the fish fully recovered and was moved to a separate 300 L (79 US gal) isolation aquarium. Aquarium-side monitoring continued and observations were made and recorded every 3 days, indicating that the gas emboli were resolving and the luxated lens was resorbing. At approximately 4 weeks, the gas emboli appeared to be completely resolved and the lens was significantly reduced in size (**18d**). The fish was returned to the original 35,000 L (9,245 US gal) mixed-species marine aquarium with no further complications.

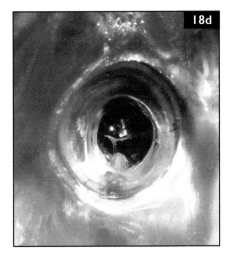

CASE 19

1 Is this a pathologic or normal finding? This is a normal finding as the anus is located within the ventral aspect of the oral cavity.

CASE 20

1 To further evaluate this case what approach would you take and what diagnostic tests would you recommend? Following an initial in-aquarium observation of the fish, noting behavior and attitude, a standard approach to medical evaluation should include a complete physical examination and visual inspection of reported lesions. This can be difficult with fish patients, especially those maintained in large aquaria. In stable patients, general anesthesia is appropriate, and often required to facilitate a thorough visual inspection and physical examination. This approach reduces the stress of handling and increases accessibility to the animal and lesions for examination. Diagnostics in this case should include microscopy of lesion impression slides or lesion swabs for cytologic evaluation. Fungal and bacterial culture with antibiotic sensitivity screening and a CBC and blood chemistry test may also be indicated. Standard diagnostics including fin biopsy, gill biopsy, and microscopy of an impression smear of scales and mucus or skin scrape should be considered to establish the general health of the fish and provide an opportunity to identify potential underlying disease or fish parasites.

Visual inspection of the anesthetized fish revealed a clear stiff needle-like foreign body protruding approximately 1–4 mm from each lesion (**20b**). These foreign bodies were manually removed and appeared to be consistent with fish

Answers

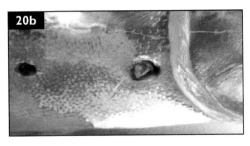

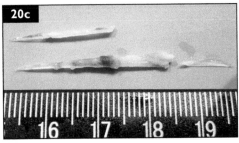

spines (**20c**). Other than the lesions and foreign bodies noted above, physical examination revealed no other abnormalities. Body condition score was reported as 2.5/5, indicating that the fish was adequately conditioned. A fecal sample collected opportunistically during anesthesia was evaluated and no ova or organisms were observed. Gills appeared healthy and no abnormal findings were reported from skin scrape microscopy. Based on findings of a foreign body, additional microscopy of lesion impression slides or lesion swabs for cytologic evaluation, fungal and bacterial culture with antibiotic sensitivity screening, or a blood collection for CBC and blood chemistry test were not performed. It was decided that a need for these diagnostics would be reassessed pending continued health status of the fish.

2 Based on your diagnostic findings how would you manage this case? Penetrating trauma with a foreign body is the most likely diagnosis in this case. The foreign body appeared to be consistent with the spine of a fish. Intraspecific and interspecific interactions or aggression are common in aquaria, especially during feeding or with reproductive maturation of fish in the system. Following removal of the spines and single application of a topical antimicrobial povidone iodine ointment, the fish was fully recovered from anesthesia and returned to the aquarium. Aquarium-side monitoring continued for approximately 2 weeks. Observations were made and recorded daily, indicating that the lesions appeared to progressively heal and were grossly undetectable within approximately 8 days.

3 What aquarium inhabitant has most likely caused this injury? On re-examination and further observation of the aquarium it was determined that one of the red lionfish exhibited minor trauma to the sheaths of tissue associated with the first three cranial spines of the dorsal fin. The distal ends or points of the first three spines matched the foreign bodies removed from the Florida pompano. It was suspected that this lionfish was involved in the interaction leading to the penetrating trauma of the pompano.

Lionfish are a venomous species that deliver neurotoxic venom to would-be predators via stiff grooved spines associated with dorsal, anal, and pelvic fins.

They are native to Indo-Pacific waters, but have been introduced and are now well established in the Atlantic Ocean, throughout the Caribbean, and along much of the eastern US coast. They were established in this aquarium as an illustration of an introduced species that does not occur naturally or until very recently has not occurred in habitats overlapping with the other common Atlantic Eastern US species of fish in the aquarium. It is possible that this novel interaction between species not normally occurring together led to this injury. The potential involvement or influence of venom on the lesion in this case is unknown.

CASE 21

1 How would you work this case up? The first step is to sedate the fish for closer examination. This was done with Aqui-S at 25 ppm. Aqui-S (a purified derivative of clove oil) was developed for humane harvesting of salmonids in New Zealand. It works very well as a sedative and anesthetic agent in both teleosts and elasmobranchs. Palpation was not helpful so ultrasonography was performed, which showed echogenic areas of irregular sizes, not consistent with eggs.

The anesthetic dose was increased to 40 ppm and an exploratory laparotomy (**21a**) was undertaken. This revealed a large red fluid-filled mass (most likely a neoplasm), which was deemed inoperable. A biopsy sample was taken for investigation (**21b**) and the surgical wound closed in two layers using simple interrupted sutures with 3/0 Maxon™ (non-cutting needle). Histopathology revealed the mass to be an undifferentiated adenocarcinoma with unknown tissue of origin. A week later the fish was euthanized.

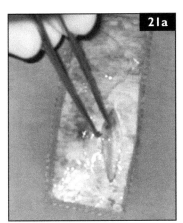
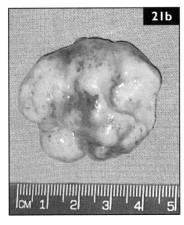

2 List your differential diagnosis. Dystocia, neoplasia, GI impaction, peritonitis, heart and/or liver failure leading to ascites.

3 **What risks are involved with this species?** Most catfish have spines on their pectoral and dorsal fins. These spines are generally not venomous but can penetrate the skin and cause injury. As such, these fish need to be handled carefully to ensure that no one is harmed.

CASE 22

1 **What conditions would be on your rule out list and which is the most likely?** Rule out list in order of occurrence: mucometra; pregnancy; ascites/coelomic effusion.

2 **What diagnostic tests would you order?** Ultrasonography. The uterus will be full of a dense proteinacious fluid called histotroph that nourishes the pups. The wall will be covered with villus trophonemata that produce the histotroph if it is a mucometra (**22b**). If gravid, there will be pups present (**22c**). If the swelling is due to ascites, there will be free fluid in the coelomic cavity and not in the uterus.

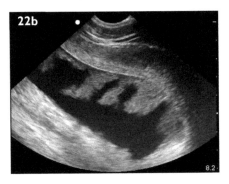

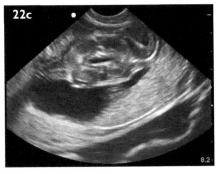

3 **If the ray is gravid, how would you explain that?** Elasmobranchs are capable of storing semen; the length of time varies by species and is not known. Parthenogenesis is a possibility.

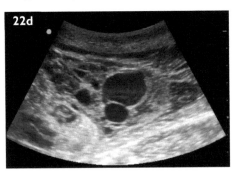

4 **What other pathologic condition usually accompanies this clinical presentation?** Rays appear to be induced ovulators and if not mated they will build up successive clutches of follicles, resulting in large cystic ovaries (**22d**).

CASE 23

1 What is the most likely diagnosis for this animal based on the impression smear? Mycobacterial organisms. Mycobacteria react positively with acid-fast stain. Mycobacteriosis is a common disease of sygnathids with *Mycobacterium marinum*, *M. fortuitum*, and *M. chelonae* being species frequently seen in aquaria. Clinical signs for mycobacteriosis include but are not limited to emaciation, growth retardation, non-healing ulcers, and granulomatous lesions.

2 What are some options that can be used to alleviate this diagnosis? There is currently no treatment published for sygnathids with mycobacteriosis. Mycobacterial organisms are ubiquitous in the environment. Known transmission routes include ingestion of the organism and direct contact with and shedding of bacteria from ulcerative lesions. Methods utilized to manage these pathogens include: (1) complete depopulation and draining then drying of the enclosure along with complete removal of substrate and exhibit items; (2) removing animals displaying clinical signs or suspected of having the disease from the system followed by euthanasia. Affected animals can act as multipliers of the disease, which then can easily overload and cause disease in immunocompetent animals within the same exhibit. Agents such as 50% ethanol and 1% benzyl-4-chlorophenol-2-phenylphenol (Lysol®) have good efficacy in killing mycobacterial organisms.

CASE 24

1 What are some differentials for the changes in the fish's appearance? Parasitic, bacterial, viral, or fungal infection, conspecific aggression, and water quality issues.

2 What diagnostics would you like to perform? The fish is anesthetized using 90 ppm MS 222 buffered with bicarbonate in order to perform another s/f/g. Results of the skin scrape and fin clip revealed numerous WBCs and a few unidentified ciliates. To treat the ciliates you decide to perform a freshwater dip for 3–4 minutes. You match the pH and temperature to the tank water and start the treatment.

CASE 25

1 What parasite is this? You think the parasite is a flatworm but are not sure, so you consult a parasitologist who tells you the parasite is *Neobenedenia*, which is a monogenean flatworm and is a common cause of cloudy eyes and skin lesions in tropical fish.

2 What treatment should be initiated? Some possible treatments for marine monogeneans include formalin, organophosphates, praziquantel, freshwater immersion, copper, hydrogen peroxide, mebendazole, fenbendazole, acetic acid, and

Answers

Chloramine T (tosylchloramide or N-chloro tosylamide). You decide to treat with 6 ppm praziquantel immersion and to repeat the treatment in 7 days. Post-praziquantel treatment you perform another examination and clear the fish from quarantine.

CASE 26

1 How did the parasite enter the system? Most likely the angelfish introduced the parasite into the system. Despite a quarantine exit examination and treatment for *Neobenedenia*, the angelfish was likely harboring some stage of the parasite that was introduced into the system and then infected other fish. Another possibility is that the parasite was already in the system and adding new fish changed the balance of the system, inducing a parasite outbreak.

2 What is the next course of action? You perform freshwater dips on a few other fish from the system and find them to be infected with *Neobenedenia*. You initiate a 4 ppm praziquantel immersion treatment q 7 days for five doses. The laboratory manager tests the praziquantel levels and discovers they are very low after only a few hours. You decide to increase the treatment to 5 ppm praziquantel q 7 days for three doses. In addition you have biologists set mesh traps on the top of the tank to screen for *Neobenedenia* eggs in order to monitor the infection in the tank. After the praziquantel treatments you perform recheck s/f/g examinations and repeat freshwater dips on several different species of fish and find no *Neobenedenia*.

CASE 27

1 What questions would you like to ask the biologists? Further information on individual history and husbandry practices would be helpful to determine which diagnostics tests should be performed. Here is a list of helpful questions (not comprehensive):

- Is the ray behaving normally?
- How are the animals fed?
- Can the biologists be sure this individual is eating?
- Where did the ray come from prior to arriving at the current institution?
- What is the ray's diet?
- Are other rays demonstrating similar signs?
- What is the water quality of the enclosure?

CASE 28

1 What diagnostic tests would you recommend? Based on the information provided you decide to perform a few diagnostic tests. The CBC and chemistry panel return as within normal limits. A skin scrape reveals no parasites and a scrape of the pectoral girdle wound reveals no infectious agents. A gill clip reveals no parasites. A coelomic aspirate is performed by introducing a 5 French red rubber catheter through the coelomic pores. The aspirate yields a light brown liquid that appears cloudy and turbid.

2 Microscopic evaluation of an aspirate reveals too numerous to count organisms of various life stages (28). What organism is this and what treatment should be initiated? The ray has a heavy burden of *Eimeria southwelli*. This is a common coccidian parasite found in both wild and managed cownose rays. Healthy cownose rays often have a mild burden of *Eimeria* and demonstrate no clinical signs. This ray was likely immunosuppressed from stress of recent collection and transport, and the *Eimeria* load was heavy enough to cause the ray to develop clinical signs of disease. Classic signs of *Eimeria* infection are dilated lymphatic vessels, eating well but not gaining weight, and the presence of turbid coelomic fluid. While it is nearly impossible to completely clear a ray of *Eimeria*, an animal diagnosed with the parasite and demonstrating clinical signs should be treated in order to reduce the parasite load. Treatments, including oral ponazuril and toltrazuril for 5 consecutive days, have been reported effective in reducing numbers of *Eimeria*. In this case, the pectoral girdle lesion was likely caused by the animal spending more time resting on the bottom due to poor body condition. Antibiotics were used to help prevent a secondary bacterial infection due to the ulcerative ventral pectoral girdle wound and appropriate nutrition was ensured by hand-feeding.

The ray was administered oral toltrazuril at 10 mg/kg PO q 24 hours for four doses. This treatment was repeated in 10 days. The ray was started on 6.6 mg/kg ceftiofur IM q 6 days for a total of four doses. Following treatment with toltrazuril the ray began to gain weight. The lymphatic vessels on the dorsal surface were no longer present and the ray appeared stronger. The animal spent less time on the bottom and over time the wound on the pectoral girdle healed.

CASE 29

1 What are your top differentials? Gravid, overweight, ascites, and coelomic mass.
2 What diagnostics do you want to pursue? Radiography and ultrasonography.
3 Once you have your diagnosis what are your treatment/management options? Radiographs are unremarkable; this is not uncommon in fish with suspected soft tissue lesions. Fat, fluid, and soft tissue have the same radiopacity, making it difficult to discern the cause of coelomic distension via radiographs. Palpation is also unremarkable; no firm mass is detected. An ultrasonographic examination reveals many 1–3 mm diameter circles (eggs) within bilateral oviducts (29). The cause for egg retention is not fully understood in aquarium maintained fish. It is due at least in part to the lack of required environmental cues for spawning,

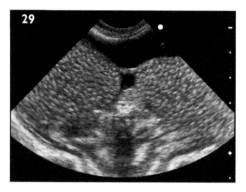

whether that is the presence of a male, appropriate nesting material, or necessary light or temperature parameters. Treatments for egg retention or dystocia in fish include manual spawning by gentle coelomic massage, Ovaprim® (salmon GnRH agonist + domperidone) administration, or ovariectomy/ovariosalpingectomy.

CASE 30

1 What are the top differentials for weight loss and scale erosion? Bacterial disease, viral disease, fungal disease, parasites, trauma.

2 What type of diagnostics would you like to perform? A skin scrape, gill clip, fin biopsy/scraping, and a fecal sample. You plan on sedating the animal in buffered MS-222 and remember reading that discus often require higher levels of anesthesia than some other freshwater fish, therefore you use a dose of 100 ppm MS-222. The skin scrape, gill clip, and fin clip reveal no parasites. To obtain a fecal sample and prime a 3 French red rubber catheter with sterile saline, insert it into the anus, infuse a small amount of saline, and then gently aspirate a fecal sample.

3 You place a fecal sample on a slide and note numerous swimming parasites (30b). What is the parasite seen on the slide? The parasites are small (5–12 × 2–13 μm), oval to tear drop shaped and swimming in a forward direction. The parasites have two visible flagella on the posterior end. You suspect the parasite to be *Spironucleus* sp. This parasite is commonly found in discus and can occur in small numbers in the GI tract of healthy fish. However, if a fish is stressed or sick, the parasites increase in number and may invade other organs and cause severe systemic disease.

4 How will you treat the fish? *Spironucleus* may be treated with metronidazole (oral and immersion), oral magnesium sulfate, and raising the water temperature for 7 days. Oral treatments appear to be most effective. You decide to treat this fish by tube feeding oral metronidazole at a dose of 50 mg/kg once daily for 5 days. The metronidazole was delivered in gruel to help the fish gain weight. Scale loss improved, the fish gained weight, and it was returned to the exhibit after a follow-up fecal sample revealed no further *Spironucleus*.

CASE 31

1 What is your presumptive diagnosis? *Glugea heraldi*, a microsporidian parasite of the subcutis in lined seahorses. *Glugea* sp. infect cells and induce hypertrophy into a xenoparasitic complex or xenoma.

2 How do you confirm your presumptive diagnosis? A milky substance exudes from lesions when ruptured by skin scrape biopsy. Microscopic examination of a squash preparation wet mount reveals a plethora of small oval spores (3.6–4.5 µm long × 1.8–2.3 µm wide), each with a large clear oval vacuole. Histologically, variably-sized xenomas cluster in the subcutis (**31b**, H&E stain, 40×, dorsal [caudal] is to the bottom of the image). Microsporidians stain Gram positive. This cross section of the seahorse tail shows the spine, epaxial and hypaxial muscle bundles, and variably-sized basophilic *Glugea* xenomas in the subcutis.

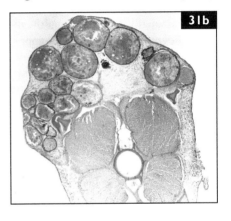

3 How will you manage the individual and the population? Microsporean infestations are unrewarding to treat. Limited success in slowing or halting disease progression for some microsporean species has been reported experimentally with toltrazuril, fumagillin, albendazole, quinine hydrochloride, monensin, and reduced temperature. For herd health purposes, preventing introduction of the parasite by quarantine is preferable. Once established, depopulation of affected and exposed individuals, followed by thorough disinfection (1,500 ppm chlorine), is required to clear an infestation reliably.

CASE 32

1 What questions do you have for the aquarist? Is the fish eating well? Is the fish male or female? How is the water quality? Do any other fish in the tank have similar clinical signs?

CASE 33

1 What stage of anesthesia is the fish exhibiting? Stage II.

2 How will you monitor anesthesia? The gill ventilation rate (GVR) is monitored closely by watching the opercula open and close. Heart rate is monitored regularly via ultrasound. The anesthetic water has an air stone to keep the DO level adequate for the procedure. If the GVR decreases or becomes sporadic, the fish will be ventilated by placing a red rubber catheter into the mouth to force water over the gills. This can be accomplished with a pump or manually with a large syringe. If the fish ceases to ventilate on its own and appears at a deep level of anesthesia, the anesthetic water can be diluted with anesthetic-free salt water.

3 What diagnostics can you perform while the fish is under anesthesia? Diagnostics can include:

Ultrasound of the coelom. This reveals a large amount of fluid. You note that the body wall is very thin, possibly from chronic fluid distension. All of the organs appear cranially displaced from the fluid. You do not note a distinct egg mass.

Radiographs. Swim bladder appears normal. Other coelomic organs are not visible on radiographs.

Coelomic aspirate. 2.5 ml of fluid were removed. The fluid is clear and has a total protein of 0.2 g/L. Cytology reveals low cellularity but there are a few rod bacteria present. Acid-fast negative.

Bloodwork. Blood is collected from the ventral midline and submitted to the laboratory. Although there are no reference range blood values for squirrelfish, based on your experience with other teleosts, you suspect that the WBC count is elevated at 55,000, and the total protein appears too low at 3.6 g/L.

4 What are your primary differentials for the coelomic distension? Chronic coelomitis (fluid accumulation) secondary to an infectious etiology, such as viral, bacterial or fungal organisms, reproductive disease, hepatic disease, renal disease, dietary hypoproteinemia, other.

CASE 34

1 What is your anesthetic plan? Since this fish was previously anesthetized at 70 ppm MS-222 and was not at a surgical plane of anesthesia, you decide to induce with 80 ppm MS-222, buffered with two parts bicarbonate to one part MS-222.

CASE 35

1 What do you do? Heart rate was detected via ultrasound and noted to be 60 bpm. You place a bifurcated tube into the oral cavity so that anesthetic water can be delivered over both sides of the gills with a pump. While the fish is not spontaneously respiring you do not want to decrease the anesthesia because the patient is mildly responsive to tactile stimulation. You decide to maintain at 80 ppm MS-222 throughout the surgery and closely monitor heart rate.

2 How do you prepare the fish for surgery? You remove a line of scales 8 cm long from the ventral midline. You gently wipe the incision site clean with a very small amount of povidone iodine. A plastic, clear drape is placed over the fish and the aquarists ensure the rest of the fish remains moist during surgery, while avoiding introducing water into the surgical field.

CASE 36

1 What, if any, samples would you like to take? Since the organs appear normal except for the ovaries you decide to perform an ovariectomy, as you suspect the abnormal ovaries are causing a coelomitis. Because the reproductive tissue and digestive tract appear similar grossly you decide to place a 5 French red rubber catheter into the digestive tract (from the cloaca) to help distinguish it from the reproductive tract. Using a hemoclip you ligate the cranial aspect of the right ovary and then place a second hemoclip at the caudal aspect. You then incise and remove the ovary. The procedure is repeated on the left ovary and both are saved for histopathology. The coelom is flushed with copious sterile saline and the skin closed with interrupted cruciate sutures using 2-0 Monocryl®.

CASE 37

1 What do you do? Continue ventilating the fish with a pump until she begins to spontaneously ventilate. Spontaneous ventilation returns within 5 minutes.
2 Given the discovery of abnormal ovaries, risk of infection, and high WBC count, what kind of post-surgical treatment is warranted? You decide to continue the enrofloxacin for three more doses every 72 hours. The incision site is examined every time the fish is handled for antibiotic administration and healing is noted. Fourteen days after surgery the sutures are removed. Biologists report that the fish started eating the day after surgery and is eating well and behaving normally, so the patient is returned to the exhibit.

CASE 38

1 Cultures and sequencing are pending, but what is the likely diagnosis? The image shows darkly pigmented fungal hyphae. The most likely cause in lumpfish is an infection with *Exophiala* or an *Exophiala*-like fungus. These are dematiaceous fungi also known as black yeast. Definitive identification requires sequencing.
2 What is the prognosis? This is an opportunistic pathogen that can infect a wide variety of aquatic and semi-aquatic organisms including invertebrates, fish, amphibians, and turtles. It can cause cutaneous, subcutaneous, and systemic infections. The infection may be chronic and is usually eventually fatal. Occasional infections by different *Exophiala* species have been reported in humans, typically following inoculation.

CASE 39

1 List some of the details about this animal's history you would like to know?
Was this fish recently caught from the wild? If not, what kind of substrate or other
material could it have been exposed to prior to arrival? Is there any history of
foreign body ingestion? Has it been defecating normally until now?

2 What should you do next? You decide to take radiographs.

3 Are there any abnormalities? There is radiodense material in the intestines, which
also appear mildly distended, and cloacal distension is also evident. The aquarist
tells you the fish had been defecating during the first week after arrival. Suspecting
a possible foreign body obstruction, you proceed with a barium contrast series, in
order to determine if the intestinal tract is obstructed.

4 Does this fish have an obstruction? This fish is not completely obstructed, as
the barium is passing through the GI tract and can be seen in the cloaca; however,
some of the barium appears to be retained within the intestine, consistent with a
partial obstruction.

The fish recovered well from the procedure and over the next week defecated
several more pieces of material, which turned out to be from a filter. Since you do
not have this type of filter in your system, the fish almost certainly ingested the
material prior to arriving at your institute. Pre-existing foreign bodies should be
considered in addition to infectious diseases when fish present with the clinical
signs noted in this case.

CASE 40

1 What are your concerns for the fish? The primary concern is water quality.
Ammonia levels will likely be elevated when the fish arrive and this can cause
severe gill irritation/damage. There are also concerns that the water temperature is
increasing and oxygen levels are decreasing.

CASE 41

1 What, if anything, can you do to help the remaining fish survive? Biologists
should acclimate the fish as quickly and safely as possible. You ask them to add
supplemental oxygen and 1 ppt salt to the tank as you have read that this species of
tetra is not sensitive to salt and you know that it will help with osmoregulation and
stress reduction. The biologists should increase the salt to 3 ppt over the next few
days. You consider adding prophylactic antibiotics to prevent secondary infections
but decide to wait to see how the fish do.

CASE 42

1 What is your next treatment plan? Unfortunately, you believe that the injury to the gills occurred during shipment due to the high ammonia. While frustrating, there is no easy way to mitigate the damage done by poor water quality. Instead, you inform the aquarists to continue with the hypersalinity treatments and supplemental oxygen, ensure the fish are eating well (offer a variety of food items if they are not eating), and maintain excellent water quality.

CASE 43

1 What would be your diagnostic plan? A thorough history reveals that this is the only fish thus affected in a large mixed species exhibit. The water quality parameters are normal and the fish is devoid of ectoparasites or other signs of disease. Based on these findings you elect to aspirate the mass and retrieve a small amount of clear fluid. The mass is not appreciably smaller after this procedure.

2 How would you manage this case? Based on your findings a decision is made to surgically resect/debulk the mass. The animal was anesthetized with 70 ppm MS-222 and the mass was lanced with a scalpel blade; a small amount of clear fluid oozed from the incision. The redundant tissue remained pronounced and was removed using forceps and scissors. Cautery was used on the areas where the cut was not crisp or where blood was evident. Several areas of the incision were left alone to give the tissue an opportunity to heal. An antimicrobial topical ointment (Derma-Vet®; nystatin, neomycin sulfate, thiostrepton, and triamcinolone acetonide) was applied to the surgical site and the fish was revived in fresh water. The resected tissue was examined under the microscope and preserved in formalin for future testing if desired. Microscopically, the tissue appeared to be thickened, possibly hyperplastic, epidermis. Several weeks after surgery, the fish appeared as shown (**43b**).

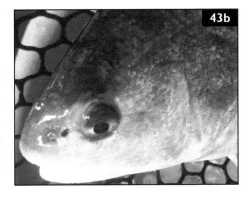

CASE 44

1 What steps should you take to work up this case? What diagnostic procedures would you like to perform? Visual examination, physical examination, radiographs. When possible it is always ideal to observe an animal in its natural environment before removing it for a hands-on examination, especially so that you can confirm that the information you are receiving is accurate and descriptive. Understanding the natural behaviors of different species will give you a great deal of information about subsequent potential abnormal behaviors.

CASE 45

1 Describe your findings. There are multiple radiolucent spots within the pouch consistent with gas bubble accumulation. The swim bladder is also enlarged caudally.
2 What are some possible reasons for this condition and what treatments can you apply? This is an example of excessive gas bubble accumulation within the pouch, tissues, and swim bladder. Gas bubble disease is often attributed to nitrogen bubble accumulation and subsequent supersaturation within tissues. Anaerobic bacteria can also produce gas that can accumulate within tissues.

A number of different treatments have been proposed and utilized with mixed success. If a system has excessive nitrogen accumulation, it is common to see multiple animals display similar clinical signs, and the environmental issue should be addressed. A minimally invasive treatment is to increase the hydrostatic pressure of the animal's environment, allowing the bubbles to shrink, although this solution may prove difficult without a deep enough system. Aspiration of the gas bubbles in the pouch can be accomplished by gently passing a 3.5 French red rubber tube into the pouch and allowing the gas to escape around and through the tube, sometimes aided by gentle manual expression or minor suction. This technique will not work if gas is present within the actual tissues. Acetazolamide (a carbonic anhydrase inhibitor) has been used as a bath, pouch lavage, or as an intramuscular injection to treat gas bubble accumulation, with mixed results reported by many individuals.

CASE 46

1 Describe the radiographic findings. The swim bladder appears to be either collapsed, filled with fluid, or filled with tissue.
2 What three basic stains can you use to help evaluate the skin lesion? Wright-Giemsa, Gram stain, and acid-fast.
3 The acid-fast stained slide is shown (46b). What is your top differential based on this result? Mycobacterial infection (numerous acid-fast positive bacilli).

CASE 47

1 What is the likely problem? This is most likely gas supersaturation, commonly known as gas bubble disease. Differentials include perimortem introduction of gas emboli (e.g. a fish dies at a surface skimmer), iatrogenic gas emboli following cutting of the primary gill filaments, and supersaturation. With multiple fish acutely affected, microbubbles in the system, and gas emboli within the capillaries, supersaturation is the most likely cause.

2 What tests could confirm your diagnosis? Confirmation requires serial measurements of total gas pressure, but a total gas pressure meter may not be readily available. An increase in DO may be appreciable using a DO meter. With either meter, it is helpful to have baseline values for the specific system.

3 List possible etiologies. Etiologies for supersaturation include:
- Air entrainment into a pump or valve.
- Increased water flow or turbulence.
- Oversupplementation by aerators, diffusers, Venturi injectors, or supersaturated well water.
- Reduced off-gassing.
- An increase in photosynthesis (e.g. a heavy algal bloom).
- An acute increase in barometric pressure.
- An acute change in temperature.

The most common etiology in a closed aquarium system is a leak in a pump or valve drawing in air under pressure, so pumps and valves should be examined first. If that is ruled out, other components of the environment and life support equipment should be examined. Any modifications to the environment or life support equipment should be monitored via clinical signs and changes in the total gas pressure.

CASE 48

1 What are some differentials for the cause of the mass and ulceration? Trauma, granuloma/abscess, neoplasia, foreign object.

CASE 49

1 In addition to radiographs, what other diagnostics or procedures could be performed while this fish is under anesthesia? Fine needle aspirate, punch biopsy with cytology and/or histopathology, surgical resection with cytology and histopathology, blood collection for CBC and chemistry.

Following radiographs, a fine needle aspirate was attempted but the mass was very solid and the aspirate was unproductive. A punch biopsy revealed osteoblasts, suggesting osteogenic activity. Blood work was unremarkable. During a second anesthetic procedure the mass was excised using electrosurgery. Histopathology (49b) revealed bony proliferation characterized by well-differentiated, acellular trabeculae forming a multilocular mass derived from both intramembranous and endochondral bone production. Due to the benign appearance, it was unclear if the

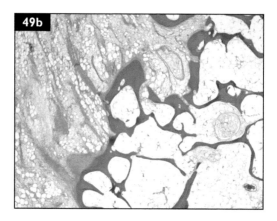

mass represented a true neoplasm of bone (osteoma), uncommon in fish, or an area of reactive hyperplasia (hyperostosis). Trauma is suspected in the development of both conditions.

CASE 50

1 What type of agent is eugenol? Eugenol is classified as a local anesthetic (like MS-222) and is the active agent in the fish anesthetic Aqui-S (10% eugenol). Eugenol can also be purchased as clove oil, although the purity and concentration of eugenol can vary. The mechanism of action of eugenol as a general anesthetic is unknown.

2 How can it be applied to fish? Eugenol is administered by immersion, as it can be absorbed via the gills. It is often used for sedation for harvest and transport, but at higher doses will produce surgical anesthesia. Recommended doses of Aqui-S are 1–5 mg/L for sedation and 15–20 mg/L for surgical anesthesia.

3 Is this compound approved for use in fish intended for human consumption? As of 2016, Aqui-S is not approved for use in the USA, but is approved for use in other countries such as Australia and New Zealand. Where approved, Aqui-S does not have any withdrawal time and can be used in fish in the food chain. In the USA, Aqui-S can only be used under an investigational new drug protocol with a 72-hour withdrawal time for fish within the food chain.

CASE 51

1 What are some potential causes for this problem? Buoyancy problems in fish can be due to a variety of reasons. The condition can be related to neural issues (e.g. spinal damage), problems with the swim bladder (e.g. bacterial, parasitic and fungal infections), neoplasia, gaseous distension of the gut, and even poor water quality (e.g. low pH, elevated nitrite).

CASE 52

1 What management and treatment options will you prescribe for nitrite toxicosis? The protocol for nitrite toxicosis is:

1 Perform 30–50% water change using a gravel siphon if appropriate.
2 Raise the salinity to 3–5 g/L (using rock salt, sea salt, aquarium salt, or pool salt) to competitively inhibit nitrite uptake.
3 Add bacteria starter culture (available from aquarium shop) to help colonize the biofilter.
4 Raise the pH to the higher end of optimal range (maintain 7.0–7.5 for oscars) to reduce the toxicity of nitrite.
5 Increase aeration since nitrite interferes with oxygenation.
6 Fast the fish for 1 week, then reintroduce food minimally.
7 Monitor nitrite (maintaining it below 0.5 mg/L with water changes).

2 How might the owner avoid this situation in future? The owner will need to be briefed on the nitrogen cycle taking approximately 4 weeks to establish in a tropical freshwater aquarium. Options owners have to avoid in this time frame include substituting the new filter material with the old one during the changeover or running the new filter and the old filter simultaneously for 1 month before dismantling the old one.

CASE 53

1 What are they and how would you treat them? These are copepods. They can be treated with trichlorfon, 0.5 ppm, for 1 hour. If the parasites do not die and drop off, the treatment can be repeated.

CASE 54

1 Describe an appropriate course of action to diagnose the problem(s). Based on presentation and ability to manually control the fish, no anesthesia was required for the initial examination. Under careful manual restraint, physical examination was performed to evaluate the eyes, oral cavity, vent, skin, fins, and gills. Ultrasonographic examination of the coelomic cavity was performed and a heart rate obtained. The fish was administered antibiotics (ceftazidime 22 mg/kg IM), glucocorticoids (prednisolone 5 mg/kg IM), antioxidants (vitamins E and C), and intracoelomic fluids (300 ml Normasol R).

Answers

CASE 55
1 What are some differentials for the cause of free air in the coelom of this fish?
Ruptured swim bladder, ruptured GI tract, full-thickness puncture to the coelom, coelomitis with gas producing microorganisms.

CASE 56
1 What is the most likely cause of the disease process in this fish? Fungal infection, specifically *Exophiala* spp.

CASE 57
1 What are these organisms and why didn't you see them before? This is the scuticociliate protozoal parasite *Uronema*. It is a free-living, opportunistic parasitic ciliate that can be found in both marine and freshwater. *Uronema* tends to be highly histophagous, causing tissue destruction and subsequently high mortality rates in fish with breaks in the skin. In this case, the *Uronema* could have been present deeper within the tissues, then multiplied significantly not long after the injury occurred. Alternatively, the organism may not have been present before, and colonized the wound after it was sustained.

2 What types of treatments are effective against this organism? A number of treatments have been proposed; however, many of these are toxic to the fish at adequate dosages. Formalin, hydrogen peroxide, malachite green, new methylene blue, chloroquine, and metronidazole have all been used with mixed success. Salinity and temperature changes, while generally safer, have yielded mixed results.

CASE 58
1 Describe the changes. There is diffuse hyperemia most apparent on unpigmented parts of the body and fins. The fins are held clamped to the body.

2 How would you remedy the situation? Fish were administered antihistamines and an alternative antibiotic was used to complete the treatment course. Although most fish do not produce histamines (including zebrafish, also a cypriniform), zebrafish have homologues for histamine receptors. The antihistamines may have blocked these receptors, explaining why the treatment was effective. Manufacturers of the florfenicol product advised using a lower dose rate (10 mg/kg) in the future.

CASE 59
1 Is there a problem? This is a pregnant male and the red bubbles are eggs. Sea dragons possess an amazing courtship dance and the female transfers the eggs to

the ventral aspect of the male's tail, where they reside for 42 days at 18°C (64.4°F) before hatching. At a few days of age the fry are about 1 cm in length (59b). They grow rapidly when fed on live day-old *Artemia* and grow about 1 cm per week for the first month.

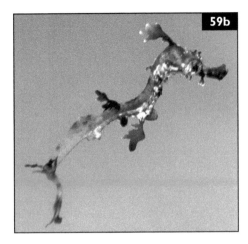

CASE 60

1 What would be most the pertinent questions to ask? You require more detail on the exhibit and its inhabitants. You also want to know how long the problem has existed.

- Is the fish eating? If so, what, and how often?
- Is the food a floating or a sinking type?
- What is the volume of the exhibit?
- What are the water quality parameters?
- Is this the only fish affected and are there other animals in the system?
- Is the trout wild caught or hatchery raised?
- Has any spawning activity been noted?
- Do guests have access to the exhibit and can they feed the fish?

2 What examination technique would you recommend? The least invasive and least costly diagnostic procedure is to physically palpate the area. The next step would likely be radiography and/or ultrasonography.

You learn the fish is eating and behaving normally and there are several other rainbow trout with the same condition. There has been no recent change in the mixed floating and sinking diet offered to the fish. The fish is removed from public display and anesthetized with 50 mg/L MS-222. Once sedated it is immediately determined that the issue is some type of hard material in the stomach. After further discussion with the aquarists you learn that salmonids are notorious for consuming foreign objects, including coins, gravel, and bark, and just weeks prior to case presentation it is learned that children had been observed throwing small pebbles from one of the lower pools to fish in the upper pool. One specific animal has had repetitive health issues and can no longer be kept on display.

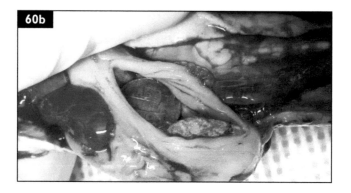

It is decided to sacrifice this animal for a full necropsy. Multiple rocks and a coin are found in the stomach (60b).

CASE 61

1 How would you manage the remaining affected trout from Case 60? Since salmonids have a simple digestive tract it is decided to try a non-invasive method to remove the foreign bodies. An instrument called an esophageal foreign body forceps (83 cm shaft), with a maximum jaw gap of 30 mm, was employed (61a).

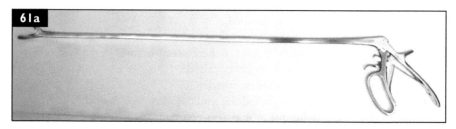

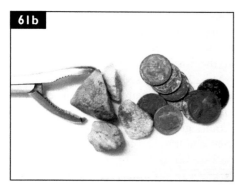

The fish was removed from public display and anesthetized as in Case 60. The fish was held at a 35° angle with the head up. The forceps were gently inserted, jaws closed, into the stomach. The forceps were gently opened when an object was detected and the object grasped. Slow removal of the forceps revealed an irregularly shaped stone that matched those in the exhibit (61b).

Repeated procedure found several more stones and multiple coins (**61c**). The fish recovered well and was returned to the exhibit without incident. Radiography could be used to confirm the removal of all foreign bodies.

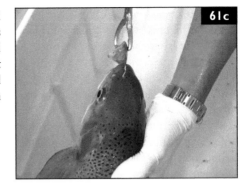

CASE 62

1 What are the skin lesions and what are their significance? The generalized lesions are the beginnings of bacterial fistulas. They indicate the shark is likely septic.

2 What would be your rule out list? (1) Septicemia secondary to egg retention metritis; this is one of the most common causes of morbidity in display female sand tiger sharks. (2) Septicemia secondary to a perforated viscous induced peritonitis. (3) Septicemia, etiology unknown.

3 What diagnostic tests would you order? A CBC and chemistry panel would be useful but an ultrasonographic examination of the uterus is diagnostic (**62c**).

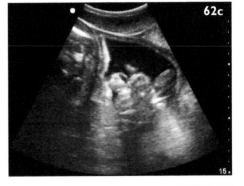

4 How would you treat this case? The treatment of choice is to sedate the shark, manually dilate the cervix, and lavage both uterine horns to remove the putrefying retained eggs (**62d**). The shark should be placed on parenteral antibiotics.

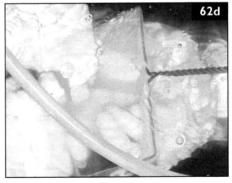

Answers

CASE 63

1 What agents would you consider? Analgesia needs should be assessed separately from anesthesia since once the anesthetics are removed their effects to block pain are removed. Fish have mu-opioid receptors and morphine has been shown to be analgesic. Fish also have a well-developed inflammatory pathway and NSAIDs (e.g. ketoprofen) have been shown to decrease inflammation and produce analgesia.

2 What are the advantages and disadvantages of each? Morphine is relatively inexpensive and effective, but is a controlled drug that requires special ordering, record keeping, and secure housing. Ketoprofen is not controlled, and is also inexpensive, but the analgesic effects may be less than morphine for acute pain (pain not from inflammation).

3 The client is looking for ways to minimize cost and asks your colleague if pain medications are needed; he has read that fish do not feel pain. How would you address this topic? Fish have all the neuroanatomic features (nociceptors, a 3-chain sensory nerve pathway, and a higher brain structure) needed to feel pain. Additionally, fish demonstrate repeatable emotional responses (e.g. avoidance, loss of normal behaviors) to pain, which are attenuated when provided analgesics. Therefore, fish should be afforded analgesics the same way other animals are.

CASE 64

1 What breed of goldfish is this? Pearlscale.

2 Identify the growths. It is not an uncommon presentation in this breed. The masses are epithelial lined and filled with clear, colorless fluid. The cysts do not normally pose a problem when small, but if they become large enough they can interfere with swimming or can tear and predispose the fish to infection. Growths can be easily removed without complication.

CASE 65

1 What is this parasite? This is *Tegastes acroporanus*, commonly known as 'red bug.'

2 What is the host range? It is a harpacticoid copepod that feeds and lives on *Acropora* corals.

3 What is the most common treatment used to control this parasite? Milbemycin oxime (Interceptor®, Novartis) has been used with success. The dose is often reported as 16 µg/L as an 8-hour immersion repeated every 7 days for three treatments. Note that while this drug is approved for use in dogs its use on corals and other invertebrates or fish is off-label.

CASE 66

1 What is this parasite? This is a species of *Neobenedenia*, a monogenean flatworm from the family Capsalidae. Features of adult *Neobenedenia* include a large, oval body, round posterior haptor, and wide smooth hamuli. The most common species is *Neobenedenia melleni*, but identification to species level is not possible from this image. The triangular structures are the eggs, which often become entrapped in the gills.

2 What is the significance of this parasite? This monogenean has a wide host range that includes species from more than 30 saltwater fish families, particularly Acanthuridae, Chaetodontidae, and Labridae. Once introduced into a system, it can be very hard to eradicate. It is a common cause of recurrent morbidity and mortality in large marine systems. It is important to prevent this parasite from getting into a naïve system.

3 What treatment options would you consider? Isolation of the affected system is critical to prevent further spread and should be routine in a quarantine system. Treatments that have shown effectiveness against adult and larval *Neobenedenia* include praziquantel immersion, organophosphate immersion, and freshwater dips. Increasing DO and providing antibiotic coverage may improve success rates if clinical signs are present. It is also important to reduce other stressors (e.g. copper therapy, social stressors). Eggs are resistant to treatment, and the maximum time that eggs remain viable is not known, so long-term pulse therapies and extensive monitoring are recommended.

CASE 67

1 What type of agent is MS-222? Tricaine methanesulfonate (MS-222) is classified as a local anesthetic drug. However, it is commonly used in fish and other aquatic species as a general anesthetic. It is approved by the US Food and Drug Administration for anesthesia is fish, crustaceans, and cold blooded aquatic animals with a 21-day withdrawal time for animals in the food chain. Although MS-222 has been used successfully in many aquatic species, the mechanism of action as a general anesthetic remains unknown.

2 Is this compound acidic or basic and how would you bring a stock solution close to neutral? Tricaine with a sulfur side chain (sulfonate) is acidic and clinically relevant solutions are acidic compared with fish. Therefore, it is recommended that when reconstituted, the solution should be buffered with an equal amount of sodium bicarbonate ($NaHCO_3$). Stock solutions are often created at 10 g/L, which would be buffered with 10 g of $NaHCO_3$ (some workers buffer as high as 1:2 MS-222:$NaHCO_3$). Typical induction doses of MS-222 range between 100 and 200 mg/L.

Answers

3 **What handling precautions should be taken and is this compound dangerous to humans?** There is little evidence this drug is toxic to humans; however, normal chemical safety should be observed such as wearing gloves and goggles and limiting exposure to skin and mucous membranes. Stock solutions should be protected from light and discarded after 3 months or if the solution becomes discolored.

4 **Does MS-222 have analgesic properties?** In order to answer this question, the reader must consider the different properties this drug might have in the body. As a local anesthetic, MS-222 would decrease nerve conduction and might provide some analgesia at the site of action. As a general anesthetic, it is unlikely to interfere with the pain pathway, but more likely just makes the brain 'sleep.' Regardless, once a fish is removed from the MS-222 solution any of those analgesic effects will be rapidly lost, so analgesia should be provided by a different mechanism such as an NSAID (ketoprofen) or opioid (e.g. morphine).

CASE 68

1 **How would you diagnose the problem and what are some possible etiologies?** The appropriate diagnostic would be a skin scraping from the bell. It can be taken by gently dragging the end of a slide or coverslip across the affected area. Tissue acquired should be examined as a wet mount then stained with a Wright's stain and a Gram stain. Two major rule outs are 'bacterial melting disease' and a ciliate infestation. Treatment would consist of baths with appropriate antibiotics such as 1-hour enrofloxacin at 5 mg/L daily. For ciliates, 3-hour metronidazole baths at 5 mg/L q 48 hours for three treatments. If necessary these drugs can be administered simultaneously.

CASE 69

1 **What would you do to examine further and make a diagnosis?** In order to examine the shark properly, it was sedated with Aqui-S at 30 ppm, and the DO level was raised to between 120 and 130% using pure oxygen and an airstone. Examination revealed a herniation of the spiral colon through the right abdominal pore. The abdominal pore is an opening from the exterior into the abdominal cavity of elasmobranchs. It is also known as the coelomic pore or equalization pore. The function of the abdominal pore is unknown but it may be involved in the excretion of acid–base ions to assist with acid–base regulation.

2 **How would you resolve the problem?** The hernia was reduced revealing a very enlarged abdominal pore opening. The abdominal pore size was decreased with simple interrupted sutures. The suture material used was 3-0 Prolene® with a semi-curved 19 mm cutting needle (**69c**).

The shark was given a prophylactic course of the antibiotic florfenicol (40 mg/kg). This injection was given intramuscularly, in the dorsal mid-body musculature, and repeated every 5 days for four treatments. The shark made an uneventful recovery from surgery and 12 months later was normal and showing no sign of relapse. The sutures were allowed to dissolve.

3 What sex is this shark? The shark is a male as there are two claspers (**69b**), one on either side of the prolapse. The claspers are a modification of the pelvic fin in sharks and are used during copulation to transfer semen into the female. The male uses only one at a time to inseminate the female during the mating process.

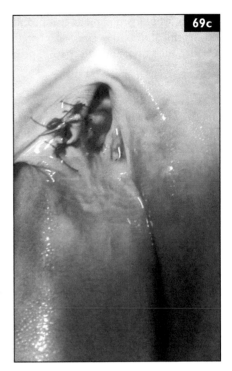

CASE 70

1 What is it? This is an *Ichthyobodo* sp. Many parasites in octopuses are symbiotic. However, *Ichthyobodo* has been associated with inflammation to the gill epithelium, and should be considered as a differential for dyspnea and tachypnea in a giant Pacific octopus.

CASE 71

1 Describe the physical examination findings present. Gas emboli in the skin between the fin rays of the dorsal fin.

2 What is your diagnosis? Gas supersaturation, 'gas bubble disease.'

3 Name potential causes for this condition. When gases are forced into water under pressure, supersaturation of the water can occur. Possible causes include Venturi injectors, faulty pumps, rapid heating of cold water, phytoplankton bloom, and certain water sources (fresh borehole water, deep wells with water that has high concentrations of either nitrogen or carbon dioxide gas).

Answers

4 How would you manage this problem? Once the source of the supersaturation is identified and addressed, surviving fish should be supported with good water quality, nutrition, and safety from predators.

CASE 72

1 To what family do spotted seatrout belong? Sciaenidae, the drum family. The common name results from their superficial resemblance to members of the Salmonidae. Spotted seatrout are popular game fish in coastal waters of the southeastern US, and are occasionally exhibited in public aquariums.

2 What is the infesting organism and what are treatment options? *Amyloodinium* sp., a parasitic dinoflagellate. The life cycle of *Amyloodinium* sp. includes a non-motile oval to pear-shaped sessile trophont phase on the host, detached reproductive cysts (tomonts), and motile flagellated infective dinospores. Lack of motility on the host sets it apart from other common protozoal ectoparasites. Diagnosis is based on microscopic findings of variably-sized oval organisms filled with densely packed dark gray to olive-brown to golden brown food vacuoles in gill or mucus wet mount preparations (**72c**, 100×). A hold-fast organ with rhizoids anchors the organism to the epithelial surface and nutrients are extracted from multiple host cells through a stomatopode or feeding tube. The hold-fast organ is visible in favorable orientations at higher magnification (**72d**, 400×), and confirms the diagnosis when observed. Treatment options include chloroquine or copper by immersion for 2–3 weeks to kill the susceptible dinospores. Reducing salinity, reducing temperature for slowing progression of disease, or increasing temperature to speed life cycle during treatment may be helpful adjuncts but will not clear an infestation.

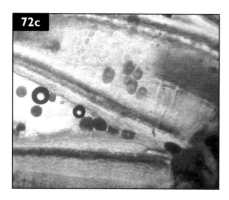

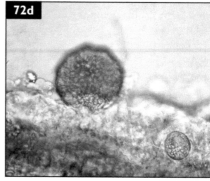

CASE 73

1 How can the sex of a giant Pacific octopus be determined? The male octopus has a modified tip to the third arm known as the hectocotylus (the reproductive portion of the third male arm; 73, arrows). This is used to transfer the spermatophores into the female's mantle.

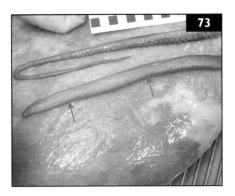

CASE 74

1 What is the common name of this condition? Head and lateral line erosion (HLLE) or hole in the head disease.

2 List possible underlying causes. The exact etiology of this syndrome is unknown. Stressors, such as overcrowding, poor water quality, or poor nutrition, may predispose fish to HLLE. Proposed causative agents include hexamitid parasites (*Spironucleus*, *Hexamita*, and *Cryptobia*), activated carbon/carbon dust, heavy metals such as copper, stray electrical voltage, ozone, UV radiation products, nutrient deficiencies of vitamins A and C and minerals, and other internal disease/stressors.

3 What are possible treatment options? Address husbandry and nutritional deficiencies. If present, activated carbon should be removed from the system. Concurrent hexamitid (*Spironucleus*/*Hexamita*) infestations should be treated with metronidazole. Some marine tropical fish HLLE cases have been successfully treated with 0.01% becaplermin (Regranex®, Ortho-McNeil Pharmaceutical Inc, Raritan, NJ). The fish is sedated and the lesions are débrided with a sterile scalpel blade and gently flushed. Regranex® is applied with sterile cotton applicators. Frequency of application varies with the severity but a single application may be sufficient. Regranex® has also been diluted with 0.9% sodium chloride to a concentration of 50% or 25%, with similar healing rates to fish treated with the full concentration.

CASE 75

1 What diagnostic tests would you undertake to make a diagnosis? A skin scrape would be the first step in establishing a diagnosis. A skin scrape involves gently scraping the lesion with a scalpel blade, scissors, or coverslip and then transferring the sample to a clean microscope slide with a few drops of seawater. You collect the skin scrape and this is what you see under the microscope (75b, 400×).

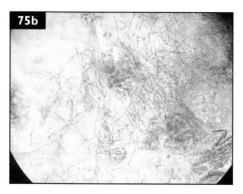

2 **What is the most likely diagnosis?** The wet preparation reveals a fungal problem, most likely the melanin-producing fungus *Exophiala* spp. *Exophiala* has emerged as a problem in many species of fish in the past decade and in particular captive sea dragons. *Exophiala* spp. are common in the environment and it would appear that stress is a factor in the development of disease.

3 **How do you treat this?** Many antifungal drugs have been tried both as baths and orally to treat *Exophiala* spp. in sea dragons, without success once clinical signs are present.

CASE 76

1 **What could this be?** It was identified as a collar of cured silicone that had come loose in the pond from one of the pipes. It was easily removed and there was no noticeable damage to the fish.

CASE 77

1 **What is the organism?** A turbellarian flatworm. *Paravortex* sp. has been reported from yellow tangs and other marine tropical species, and *Ichthyophaga* sp. has been reported from carangids including lookdowns. They can be found on or in the skin and occasionally gills. Turbellarians are flatworms that include mostly free-living and some parasitic species. Although sometimes confused with dactylogyrid monogeneans, turbellarians have only two eyespots (dactylogyrids have four) and are covered with cilia (dactylogyrids have none) that create a zone of turbidity at the margins of the organism. Parasitic turbellarians have a direct life cycle, with both parasitic and free-living stages.

2 **How do you treat it?** Various turbellarian infestations have been treated successfully with formalin dips and baths, osmotic stress (reduced salinity baths or freshwater dips), formalin and osmotic stress combined, or organophosphates.

CASE 78

1 **Why might that be?** Common reasons for ineffective treatments include under-dosing (recalculate the water volume and the amount of drug required), leaving ozone on or charcoal in the filter (check filtration), drug resistance, undiagnosed

concurrent disease(s), among others. In this case, the pH of the water was high (8.2, an effect of the concrete pond), causing organophosphates like trichlorfon to degrade quickly.

2 How would you manage the situation? An alternative drug, diflubenzuron at a dose of 0.1 mg/L, was applied and repeated on days 14 and 30.

CASE 79

1 What are your primary differentials for this lesion? The primary differential to consider is neoplasia. Other differentials include chronic trauma and granuloma from an infectious pathogen such as *Mycobacterium*.

2 What is your diagnostic plan for this fish? The next diagnostic step would be to take a surgical biopsy with histopathology.

CASE 80

1 Without excess skin to create a primary closure, what is the expected course of healing for the mass removal site? The site will heal by secondary intention. This is a common choice due to the non-elastic nature of fish skin. Scab formation does not occur in fish; however, epithelialization typically occurs quickly. By allowing the wound to remain open, the possibility of complications, including abscess formation and necrosis, are reduced. In this case, evidence of re-epithelialization was observed 24 hours after surgery.

2 What is the prognosis for fish with a spindle cell neoplasm? In most cases of spindle cell neoplasms the prognosis is generally good. Surgical debulking or excision is recommended, as they tend to be locally invasive, and recurrent unless excision is complete. Growth rate and metastasis are variable.

3 Why do you think the tumor recurred? The initial surgery removed the bulk of the tumor, but cryoablation left some neoplastic tissue at the margins. Removal of tumor tissue with clean margins is considered curative for most spindle cell neoplasms.

CASE 81

1 What would you do next? Biopsy for histopathology would be a good idea. Furthermore, ultrasonography and radiography would likely determine the size and depth of the lesions. Several lesions on several fish were biopsied. All of them showed only inflammatory response and in none could a specific etiologic agent be found.

2 Should you revisit the history? Yes, revisit the history. Sometimes asking several aquarists questions will result in a valuable lead. In some cases it is also best to check the actual water quality parameters yourself. In this case, the water quality was acceptable and had been stable for some time. However, while checking these

Answers

records, a note about the addition of new fish was found. The curator's boss told him to put more fish into that tank, which he did. That important bit of information was left out of the original history. They were added just a few days before the lumps were noticed. With that history the aquarist was instructed to remove some of the new fish and all of the lesions started to regress and were gone within 1 month without treatment. The suspected etiology was overcrowding causing trauma to tank mates from the spines.

CASE 82

1 What type of scale is this? Ctenoid scale (a type of leptoid or bony-ridge scale).
2 Where does a scale arise in the skin (epidermis or dermis)? From a scale pocket in the dermis.
3 Name other common types of scales and provide examples of species that have that type of scale.
- Cycloid scales are another type of leptoid/bony-ridge scale (in the same group as ctenoid scales), have a smooth outer edge, and can be found on fish such as salmon and carp.
- Placoid scales – cartilaginous fish.
- Ganoid scales – gars (family Lepisosteidae) and bichirs (family Polypteridae)
- Cosmoid scales – lungfish.

4 How does the epidermis differ in fish without scales? The epidermis is typically thicker in fish without scales or in areas with no scales.

CASE 83

1 What could have happened? The problem is almost certainly environment related. It was found that the water temperature rose to 36°C (96.8°F). The fish likely died from a combination of hyperthermia and hypoxia.
2 What gross signs can you observe to support the diagnosis? Observable signs for this problem may include water warmth, a heater indicator light continuously in the on position, flared opercula, and bleached gills. High water temperature can be particularly stressful for some marine fish since water with higher salinity contains less DO, assuming temperature and pressure are the same.

CASE 84

1 Identify the structures present in the stomach wall on wet mount examination. Granulomas.
2 What is the most likely causative agent? *Cryptobia iubilans.*
3 Describe the organism's appearance on light microscopy. *Cryptobia iubilans* is a small (10–13 μm long and 2 μm wide) protozoal parasite with two flagella

of unequal lengths that extend from the anterior end. Flagellated trophozoites are elongate (acute infection) to oval/tear-drop shape (chronic infection) with a characteristic slow undulating movement.

4 What findings would you expect on histopathology of the internal organs? On histology, single to coalescing acid-fast negative granulomas can be seen in the gastric mucosa or submucosa (granulomatous gastritis). In some cases, slender, elongate, ovoid flagellated trophozoites can be found within vacuoles of the macrophages or within the gastric epithelium. Granulomas can also be found in other organs, including the liver, spleen, mesentery, mesenteric fat, heart, swim bladder, anterior and posterior kidneys, gall bladder, ovary, brain, and eye.

5 What is required for definitive diagnosis? Species identification requires electron microscopy.

6 What are the treatment options? There is no current know effective treatment for *Cryptobia iubilans* in cichlids. Due to the granulomatous gastritis caused by the parasites it is nearly impossible to completely eradicate. Attempts to treat affected fish have resulted in little to no response. Some farmers have reported decreased mortalities with sulfa drugs (e.g. sulfadimethoxine), but this may just help with secondary infections or co-infections. Treatments with dimetridazole and 2-amino-5-nitrothiazol have showed reduction of the prevalence of *C. iubilans* in experimentally infected fish but more studies are needed to develop treatment recommendations. Appropriate quarantine procedures are helpful in preventing introduction.

CASE 85

1 What would your differentials be for the lesions seen on this yellow perch (*Perca flavescens*) (85a)? Some type of encysted parasite should be at the top of your list. Bacterial or fungal granulomas would be next, followed distantly by neoplasia and foreign body.

2 What diagnostic tests would you perform to arrive at a diagnosis? Biopsy and/or fine needle aspirate would likely yield a diagnosis. If the fish was a necropsy candidate, then a full post-mortem gross and microscopic examination would be in order. In this case, aspiration of a periocular nodule (xenoma) produced numerous spores with paired polar filaments indicating this is a myxosporidian metazoan parasite (**85b**; Diff-Quik® stain, 10×).

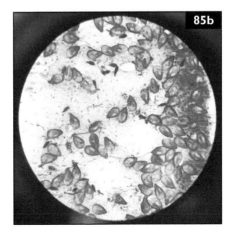

Answers

These organisms require an intermediate host and a chemotherapeutic option is currently lacking.

CASE 86

1 When is assist feeding indicated? Candidates for intubation feeding include clinically ill animals, animals exposed to prolonged transportation time, new acquisitions, and in some cases newborns. Assist feeding should be performed when the animal stops feeding or when noticeable loss of body mass and physical manifestations of malnutrition and/or dehydration are observed.

2 How can tube assist feeding be implemented and what should be fed? Sedation is usually not necessary. Tonic immobility, which is a non-chemical restraint technique, can be used with most elasmobranchs. If necessary, anesthetic agents can be considered. A food mixture of freshly-peeled prawns and mussel meat (at a 2:1 ratio), vitamin B complex, and fresh garlic blended in drinking water (~25–50% of the total mixture) is recommended. Commercial elasmobranch gel food mixture can be used as well. An appropriate diameter and length of feeding tube is selected based on the size of the animal and its anatomy (**86a, b**) and preloaded with the food mixture to minimize air pockets. The lubricated feeding tube is carefully and slowly inserted into the mouth and esophagus to the stomach. Care must be taken not to push the tube too far. Food is then passed

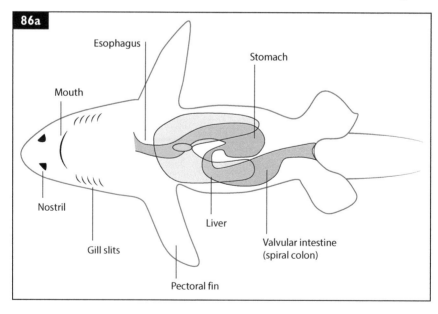

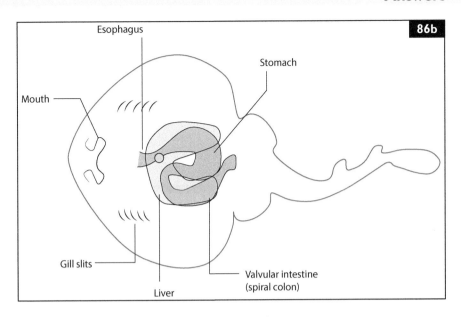

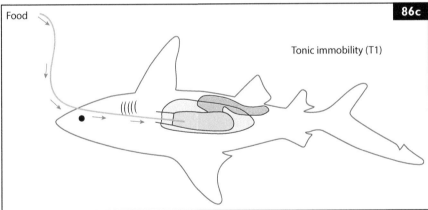

directly into the stomach (**86c**). Elasmobranchs should receive approximately 1% of body weight and frequency depends on the clinical signs and compliance.

CASE 87

1 How would you manage the situation? These growths arise from around the head/face and do not invade the eye. This fish was anesthetized in a bath with alfaxalone at 5–6.0 mg/L. A scalpel blade was used to shear off the excess growth

Answers

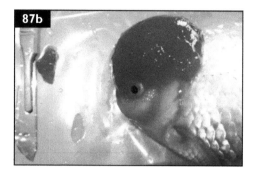

87b

taking care not to damage the eyes (**87b**). Dilute Betadine® (povidone iodine) (1 part Betadine®: 9 parts saline) was applied topically on the exposed surface and the fish given flunixin at 0.3 mg/kg IM for pain management.

CASE 88

1 What is the problem? The gills are displaying severe hyperplasia (thickening) of the secondary lamellae. Many of the secondary lamellae are fused. This usually occurs as a result of chronic inflammation. Severe hyperplasia like this dramatically

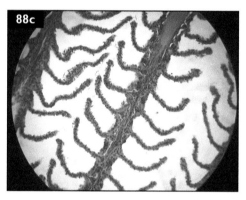

88c

decreases the surface area, resulting in poorly efficient gills with reduced oxygen absorption, carbon dioxide elimination, and ammonia excretion. Normal gill morphology is shown (**88c**).

2 What are the possible causes? There are two main causes of gill hyperplasia. The first is secondary to water quality problems and the second is a response to external pathogens such as bacteria or monogeneans (gill flukes). The wet preparations of the Murray cod gills and the histopathology did not reveal any pathogens, so a water quality problem was suspected.

The standard water parameters were all within normal range. This included temperature, pH, ammonia, nitrite, and nitrate. On further investigation, it was discovered that the previous summer the aquarist maintaining the tank had placed the tank on a slow flow through of fresh water to assist in maintaining water temperature. However, the water was straight from the tap, and had not undergone any pretreatment. A low-grade, chronic chlorine toxicity was suspected as the cause of the gill damage. This problem was corrected, the fish recovered, and its normal appetite returned.

CASE 89

1 What are the two large radiolucent structures in the center of the image? The swim bladder.

2 Are these normal? Yes. In goldfish the swim bladder is a double-chambered organ located dorsally within the body cavity.

3 How is radiography of this organ useful? Buoyancy is controlled by the amount and distribution of free gas within the body, most of which is enclosed within the swim bladder. Buoyancy disorders are common in goldfish, and radiography is the most effective means of identifying abnormalities. The anterior chamber has a thick tunica externa that is firmly attached to the Weberian ossicles and a flattened bony process at the base of the fourth vertebra. This is a useful landmark since fluid filling the anterior chamber can render it 'invisible' in the homogeneous radiodensity of the intracoelomic tissues. The posterior chamber connects to the anterior chamber by a short narrow duct and to the proximal esophagus by the long patent pneumatic duct. This chamber has no thick tunica and can vary significantly in size between different goldfish varieties, occasionally over-inflating or rupturing in some cases. The lack of any direct attachment to the skeleton allows the posterior chamber to deviate horizontally and ventrally following enlargement of surrounding organs. The posterior kidney is located dorsally between the two chambers of the swim bladder and enlargement can result in an increased separation of both chambers or displacement of the posterior chamber. Over- and under-inflation of the chambers can also be identified, although this requires experience to interpret. Both lateral and dorsoventral radiographs should be taken, and a horizontal beam view in cases where fluid is present within the swim bladder.

CASE 90

1 What questions would you like to ask the owners? Questions that will help you find the correct diagnosis include:

- Have you seen Goldie flashing? (Ectoparasites causing pruritus that can lead to self-trauma.)
- What substrate do you use in the tank? (Some substrates can be swallowed, leading to GI obstruction or impaction.)
- Do you have any sharp objects in the tank? (Decorations with sharp edges can injure fish.)
- Are there any other fish in the tank?
- Are they displaying similar symptoms? (Is this a system-wide problem or an individual problem?)
- Are there signs of aggression among the fish?

Answers

2 **What else would you like to do?** A physical examination of the sedated fish and an in-depth exploration of the inflamed area are recommended. The gills on both sides are normal in appearance. Opercular movements are equal and show no abnormalities. An oral examination reveals an oval object in the pharynx (**90b**). Kelly forceps were used to grasp the object (**90c**), which turned out to be a piece of gravel lodged in the pharynx, creating an obstruction. A course of injectable enrofloxacin was started and 0.1% salinity recommended for a week to reduce osmotic stress and improve healing.

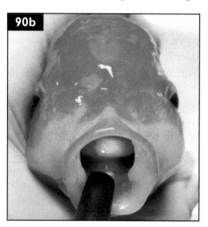 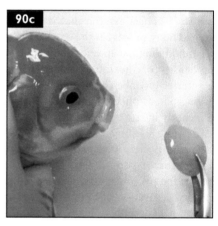

A follow-up phone call with the owner 1 week later revealed Goldie was completely back to normal, eating well, and moving throughout the water column.

CASE 91

1 **Suggest a course of action and possible diagnosis.**

Diagnostics:

- Under anesthesia, examine the most affected fish for gill disease and subtle clinical lesions (e.g. hyphema).
- Take scrapings from the skin and gills and microscopically examine wet preparations.
- If possible, sacrifice a moribund fish, perform a necropsy, sampling all the major organs for histologic examination, namely the gills, heart, liver, GI tract, anterior and posterior kidneys, spleen, brain, and any visible lesions.
- Take bacteriological swabs from the posterior kidney using aseptic technique.

- Send fresh samples of anterior and posterior kidney, spleen, and gill in transport medium on ice to a suitable fish laboratory for conventional and molecular virology. Gill samples in 90% industrial methylated spirit or 70% ethanol are also useful.

Initial therapy:
- Change 30% of the water in the pond.
- Add sodium chloride (salt), increasing salinity to 2.5–5.0 ppt.
- Remove excess aquatic weeds and use fountains, air pumps with air stones, or diffusers to improve oxygenation of the water.
- Use appropriate anti-parasitic therapy depending on results from the wet preps.
- Start antibiotic therapy by injecting the worst/anorexic fish and medicating the feed.

In this case, there were no visible lesions and no response to antibiotics. The clinical history and lower water temperature suggested that the fish had 'koi sleepy disease' due to a pox-like virus (carp edema virus), an infectious disease that occurs between 12 and 15°C (53.6 and 59°F). A water heater was fitted and the temperature increased to 18°C (64.4°F). Histologic examination revealed significant proliferative changes in the gills and virology tests were positive for carp edema virus. There was a dramatic improvement after the water temperature increased. There were no mortalities and no relapse of disease when the temperatures decreased the following winter. At present koi sleepy disease has been confirmed in Europe and Japan. In severe cases, there can be skin erosions, sunken eyes, and a chronic mortality of up to 70%. There is no effective treatment but raising the water temperature above 15°C (59°F), and improving aeration, are beneficial. Antibiotics should be given to prevent secondary bacterial disease since it may take several weeks for koi to recover.

CASE 92

1 Why is this, and how would you manage the situation? Copper sulfate is contraindicated in certain fish species, including clownfish, elasmobranchs, and syngnathids. In the event of copper toxicity, management involves immediately replacing the water in the hospital tank with water from the main aquarium, employing activated charcoal, and adding EDTA at a rate of 30 mg/L to bind the copper. These fish recovered almost immediately.

CASE 93

1 What abnormality can you identify on this piece of moon coral (*Favia* sp.) (93) and list various possible causes? The live brown coral tissue at the bottom of the image has died and left necrotic gelatinous matter within the polygonal calices (concave depressions housing the polyps), exposing the underlying white coral skeleton. The bright green central oral disc of the polyp is normal in this nocturnal species and fluoresces under UV light.

There are many causes of localized areas of coral necrosis but most are poorly documented and often the result of several factors. Koch's postulates have yet to be proven for most infectious agents. Common causes of polyp death include:

- Rough handling, drying out during shipping, or prolonged contact with the transport bag surface or ice in the packing container.
- Poor water quality due to high levels of ammonia, nitrite, nitrate, phosphate; high pH and salinity; low levels of DO; low pH and salinity.
- Poor positioning in the aquarium with damage caused by strong direct current (e.g. too close to the powerhead); poor light exposure; sedimentation; stinging by being positioned too close to aggressive corals.
- Infectious disease agents such as bacteria (e.g. *Vibrio* spp.), ciliate parasites, and some blue–green algae.

CASE 94

1 What abnormalities can be identified? The posterior chamber of the swim bladder is displaced ventrally on the lateral view and displaced laterally to the right side on the dorsoventral view. There is no obvious fluid in either chamber and no excess gas in the bowel.

2 What is the most likely cause of the problem? Enlargement of one or both sides of the posterior kidney, which is located dorsally between the two chambers of the swim bladder. This is a common problem in goldfish and may be due to polycystic changes (a developmental anomaly or following infection with the myxosporidian parasite *Hoferellus carassii*), extensive granulomata, or neoplasia.

3 How can this be confirmed? An ultrasound scan will identify the nature of the swollen tissue and determine if it is cystic or solid. In this case, the displacement was due to polycystic kidney disease affecting the left kidney (**94c**), although no parasites were found on histologic examination of kidney biopsies.

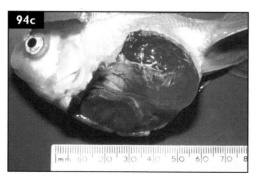

4 What treatment do you suggest? There is no known treatment for this chronic condition that can cause substantial and often asymmetrical abdominal swelling. Fish can survive for many months before developing clinical problems as the swelling becomes more pronounced; they should be euthanized when secondary complications (e.g. deep skin ulceration) occur.

CASE 95

1 Is there significance to the sudden behavior change in all of the fish? It is not uncommon for pond owners to report most of their fish are 'hiding' or are at the bottom of the water column after a predator attack.

2 What are possible causes for an increased opercular rate (essentially an increased respiratory rate)? Any disease that directly affects the gills (e.g. koi herpesvirus, parasitism, bacterial gill disease, high turbidity levels, etc.), poor water quality parameters affecting respiration (nitrite toxicity, reduced DO, rapid pH changes, elevated ammonia levels, elevated hydrogen sulfide levels), and some systemic diseases (especially those leading to anemia, sepsis) can cause increased opercular movements. In addition, increased stress levels (e.g. capture or predation attempts) can also result in an increased respiratory rate.

CASE 96

1 What is the most likely cause of these lesions? A raccoon was recently observed in the neighborhood by the owner and several neighbors. Raccoons are one of the many predators of pond fish. Other predators include mink, herons, domestic pets, ospreys and other birds of prey. Although there were no witnesses to the event, the most likely scenario is an attempted grabbing of the fish by the raccoon. The fish was able to escape, most likely due to her large size and weight. The depth and width of the grooves on the body wall are consistent with the nails of a raccoon.

2 How would you approach treatment? The treatment in this case consisted of débriding the area of necrosis, systemic antibiotic therapy, analgesic medication, and prevention of further predation. Following débridement of the necrotic tissue, ceftazidime 20 mg/kg IM q 72 hours was initiated and a single injection of carprofen 1 mg/kg IM was also given. A recommendation for the use of 0.1% non-iodized salt added to the pond was also made to help improve healing and as a general osmotic stress reducer.

To help reduce workload by the owner and capture stress on the fish, a mesh cage was assembled to allow Sunshine to remain in the pond (eliminating the need for a hospital tank) but still be accessible for treatments. The pond was then covered with netting stretched over a polyvinyl chloride frame to prevent further predator attacks (**96d**). A recheck 2 weeks later showed 90% improvement in the gill lesions and

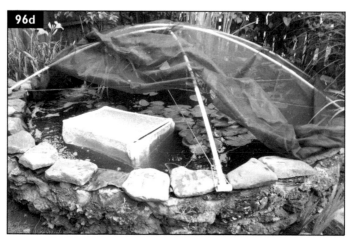

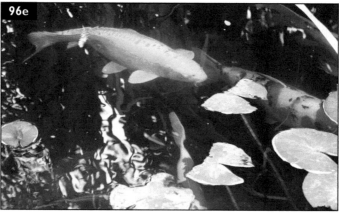

Sunshine was starting to eat. She was released from the mesh cage into the general population. A follow-up phone call 1 month after initiating treatment revealed she was back to normal behavior and appetite (**96e**).

CASE 97

1 Name the structure pictured here that is being sampled for bacterial culture and sensitivity in an adult koi. Posterior kidney.

2 Describe the physiologic function of this structure and how it differs from the other part of this organ. The posterior (caudal) kidney contains the excretory components responsible for excretion of nitrogenous wastes and osmoregulation. The anterior (cranial) kidney is predominantly hematopoietic.

CASE 98

1 What abnormality can you identify on this fragmented piece of pineapple coral (*Favia* sp.) (98)? Green and red filamentous algae are visible growing on both sides of this piece of coral. The algae are growing on areas where coral has died and the underlying calcium carbonate skeleton has been exposed.

2 What effect does this have in marine reef systems? Algae can grow rapidly in nutrient-rich water and overwhelm the coral, reducing the light reaching the essential zooxanthellae in the live coral tissue. Algal overgrowth often results in stress to the inhabitants through hypoxia and pH changes due to algal respiration at night.

3 How would this problem be controlled? Algal growth is encouraged by high levels of nitrate and phosphates in the water. These are reduced by using water produced by reverse osmosis since tap water often has high levels of these nutrients. Nitrogen-removing resins can also be used in combination with a 'phosphate sponge' (ferric hydroxide), a granular compound that absorbs phosphate from the water supply. The salt used to produce the seawater should be formulated for reef systems that contain invertebrates rather than fish-only systems. Overfeeding with decomposition of organic matter liberates phosphate into the system. The use of low-grade activated carbon can also be a source of phosphate. An 'algal scrubber' or refugium, a separate tank containing macro-algae (seaweed) that is illuminated at night, can be built into larger reef systems to reduce available nutrients from the water. Protein skimmers and ozone can also remove algal nutrients. Once established, filamentous algae must be removed manually, although herbivorous fish, snails, and crabs can also be used. Free-floating unicellular algae can be controlled using UV sterilization and a filter sock that mechanically removes particles down to 100 microns in size.

CASE 99

1 What are your differential diagnoses? Differentials include neoplasia, thyroid hyperplasia (goiter), bacterial or fungal granuloma, encysted parasite(s), and foreign body.

2 What is your next step? A routine examination including skin scrapes, gill clips, fin clips, and blood work is unremarkable. The only problems noted are the branchial masses and the HLLE. While not employed here, endoscopy can be valuable for exploring the branchial chamber. The plan was to obtain a fine needle aspirate (FNA) and then biopsy if warranted. The FNA sample was placed on several slides and stained with Wright's stain, Gram stain and an acid-fast stain. The acid-fast stain revealed countless acid-fast rods consistent with *Mycobacterium* spp. (thus a mycobacterial granuloma). The curator decided to allow this fish and others in the same system to live out their lives but to quarantine the system. This particular fish lived for about 2 more years. It should be noted that without a biopsy and histopathology concurrent goiter cannot be ruled out.

151

Answers

CASE 100

1 How would you manage this situation? It is not unusual to find more than one type of ectoparasite. To eradicate the skin fluke, but preserve the anchor worms, a targeted approach is necessary. In this situation, the fish were treated with a single immersion dose of praziquantel at a rate of 5.0 mg/L.

CASE 101

1 What causes would be included on your differential diagnosis list? The most common cause of a corneo-conjunctival mass is an inflammatory reaction. Inflammatory lesions can result from infectious agents such as viruses, bacteria, and fungi. Another possible cause of this condition would be a corneal neoplasm.

2 What diagnostic tests would you perform to determine the cause of the problem? After the patient was properly sedated with 70 ppm MS-222 immersion the mass was swabbed and biopsied. Only partial surgical removal was accomplished due to the corneal and conjunctival attachments. Cytologic evaluation of an imprint made from the biopsied tissue revealed squamous epithelial cells and a significant number of white blood cells. No lipid or free proteinaceous material was observed and no bacterial or fungal organisms were found. The long-acting

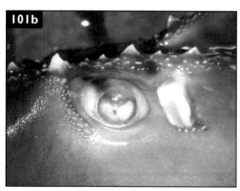

antibiotic ceftiofur (6.6 mg/kg) was administered via intramuscular injection. The biopsied tissue was placed in 10% formalin and submitted for histopathology. The histopathology findings revealed a mass of inflammatory and red blood cells. No neoplastic cells were observed and the bacterial culture was negative. After 4 weeks the mass disappeared and the eye completely healed (**101b**). There was no recurrence of the mass.

3 What is the cause of this lesion? This corneo-conjucntival mass was not neoplastic based on the histopathology results. The corneal epithelial cells likely produced the inflammatory and hyperplastic reaction in response to a traumatic injury, most likely incurred during the quarantine process.

CASE 102

1 What is the name of the missing structure of the left eye? The structure not visible in the left eye is called an 'operculum.'

2 **What elasmobranchs have such a structure?** The operculum is present in batoid rays (Batoidea – skates and rays).

3 **What is the purpose of this structure?** It is believed the operculum helps focus images in low light.

4 **What might have happened and what would you do?** It turns out this was a rambunctious young animal that may have bumped into one of the other bowmouth guitar fish in the holding tank. The first thing to do when seeing something new and/ or odd is to contact colleagues that might have dealt with this before. In this case, such efforts were unrewarding, and after examination with an ophthalmoscope, the clinician felt the operculum had flipped and rolled up. A decision was made to flush it back into place without touching it. Using general and topical anesthesia, fluid was removed from the anterior chamber, while a stream of sterile saline was used to flush the operculum (**102c, d**). This technique worked and approximately equal volumes of fluid were removed and added. Topical antibiotics were also applied to the affected eye. After several hours the eye looked normal and remained that way.

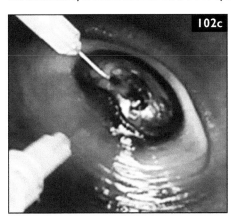 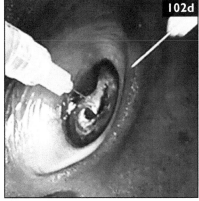

CASE 103

1 **What is precopulatory behavior?** Precopulatory behavior is an aggressive interaction where the male engages the female with its teeth. In this case, the male zebra shark followed the female and bit vigorously at her pectoral fins and distal tail. At one point the female was turned on her back and both sharks remained motionless for several minutes (**103b, c**). Tail injuries on mature female zebra sharks resulting from precopulatory behavior are not uncommon. If an injury is minor, it can be left alone for self-recovery. However, medical intervention was necessary for this case to prevent sepsis, since the wound possessed necrotic tissue, which can lead to septicemia.

Answers

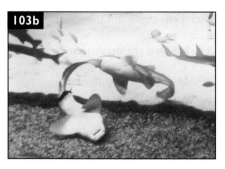

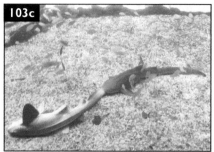

2 How would you treat this lesion? Due to the severity of the tail wound partial amputation was recommended. The animal was anesthetized with propofol at 2.5 mg/kg by slow intravenous injection. The damaged tissues were amputated with a sterile scalpel blade. Pressure with sterile gauze and styptic powder were applied to control bleeding. Post-surgical treatment with enrofloxacin at 5 mg/kg PO q 24 hours for 14 days would be warranted.

No signs of post-surgical infection were observed (**103d, e** taken 3 days after surgery). Tissue regeneration (as evidenced by granulation tissue formation and vascularization) was observed within the recovery period (**103f** taken at 7 days). At 21 days the amputation site was completely healed (**103g**), the swimming pattern was normal, and the shark had a good appetite.

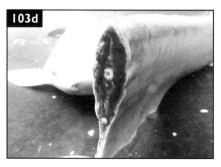

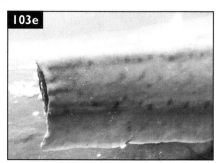

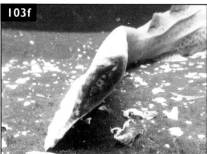

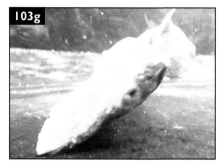

CASE 104

1 What is your recommendation for a next step? An examination and work up is the next logical step. Unfortunately, the aquarist was reluctant to catch the fish, and her hope was to empirically place the fish on oral antibiotics if/when it started to eat. A month passed and finally the eel was captured despite some major logistical challenges. It had been very difficult to see the mass while the fish was on exhibit since the eel was mostly hidden or in the dark. Once out, it was obvious the lesion was much more extensive than realized. The animal was anesthetized with MS-222 for an examination and work up including blood analysis. The mass extended through the maxilla into the mouth and to the cranial end of the rostrum. Fine needle aspirates and impression smears showed fungal organisms. The prognosis was poor, but further diagnostics were discussed in case there was an underlying cause, as well as treatments with antifungals. Due to the extensive damage already present and the fact that the animal would be very difficult to treat regularly, the curator elected euthanasia. On necropsy no other lesions were found and the final diagnosis was fungal granuloma based on the earlier diagnostics. It should be noted that if desired or warranted the mass could have been cultured or analyzed using PCR in order to attempt etiologic agent identification.

CASE 105

1 Discuss the options available. Fibromas on the eye can grow very large and become avulsed or subject to trauma from other fish or aquarium furniture. Unless owners perceive the fish to be suffering, many fish keepers only consider euthanasia as a last resort. There are no proven chemotherapeutic protocols that are effective against neoplasms in fish. Effective surgical excision of tumors is not without risk but can be rewarding, especially if surgical debulking is followed with cryo or laser surgery. The small masses noted on the body have the potential to develop into large tumors but many will remain small and of little clinical significance. Removal of the whole affected eye with the attached tumor often results in complete resolution, although there are risks and poor technique can be fatal. In this case, the eye was removed (105c) and the fish recovered uneventfully.

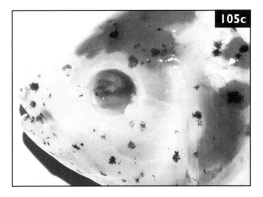

105c

The orbital socket healed well with minimal intervention following surgery. The application of dilute povidone iodine to the site followed by a waterproof dressing (Orahesive®, ConvaTec) and a single antibiotic injection was all that was required. The small masses on the skin remained the same size over the following months.

CASE 106

1 **Discuss the practicality of such a cosmetic procedure.** The insertion of prosthetic eyes has been reported in striped bass and was investigated because fish on

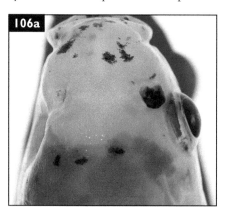 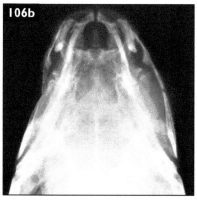

display at public aquaria are often euthanized due to their unsightly appearance following the loss of an eye. Although initially successful, long-term retention of the prosthesis beyond the end of the 8-week study was unsuccessful. There is significant remodelling of the facial bones over the following weeks after the globe is removed. This goldfish was examined 4 months later for an unrelated problem (106a) and a radiograph of the skull was obtained (106b), which shows the degree of change that can occur.

CASE 107

1 **How would you describe biological filtration?** The biological filter is the best and most efficient means of removing nitrogenous waste from an aquatic system. This type of filter utilizes nitrification, a natural process that occurs constantly in soil and water. Nitrification involves the conversion of ammonia to nitrate in a two-step process. Stable populations of microorganisms must exist in the filter for the nitrification process to perform efficiently. These microorganisms require plenty of oxygen and ammonia as a food source. Under normal conditions it takes several weeks for the filter to develop and function adequately.

2 What can happen if a biological filter is not mature? When an aquarist attempts to 'rush' the biological filter by loading a system with animals before the filter is established they will likely be confronted with 'new tank syndrome.' This syndrome is responsible for the death of countless pet fish and invertebrates each year. Patience is the key when starting a new system. Begin with a few hardy fish and then gradually add more fish (properly quarantined) over time when the filter becomes established. If an aquarist insists on a stocked aquarium in the absolute shortest period of time, there are some commercially available biological filter starter solutions that contain nitrification bacterial cultures, and may shorten the interval by a day or two. An alternative is some type of chemical filtration that physically removes nitrogen compounds from the water. A simple box filter containing activated carbon may be used to help remove some of the nitrogen load during the first few weeks that a system is operating. Care should be taken not to remove all of the available ammonia and nitrite or else there will be no 'food' for the nitrifying microorganisms.

3 Can you give some examples of biological filter types? There are several different types of biological filters. The first type is the popular undergravel filter (**107a**). Most of these filters utilize a plastic grid that lies at the bottom of the tank, allowing for a small water space beneath it. Several inches of gravel are then placed over the porous plate. Aerated water is pulled through the gravel bed via airlift tubes that are attached to the plastic grid. The nitrifying organisms become established on the grid/gravel and the aquarium water is literally pulled through the filter

bed, exposing the nitrifying bacteria to the nitrogen compounds in the water. A second type of biological filter is termed the wet/dry filter, also called an ammonia tower or trickle filter (**107b**). With these filters, the bacterial bed is not submerged in water but rather is sprayed with aerated water that passes through the filter bed by means

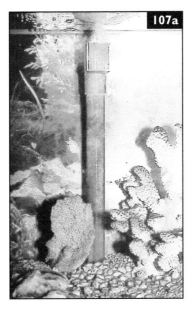 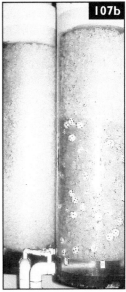

of gravity. These filters are desirable since they tend to allow for a large surface area and consequently many organisms can colonize the filter.

4 What microorganisms are involved in biological filtration? The cycling of nitrogen is primarily performed by two genera of bacteria, *Nitrosomonas* and *Nitrobacter*, and a group of microorganisms known as the Archaea.

CASE 108

1 What is the cause of this clinical signs? Septicemia is a common clinical finding in captive elasmobranchs. Antibiotic therapy and supportive care is frequently successful in such cases.

2 How would you treat this case? Ceftriaxone 30 mg/kg, diluted in 5 ml of elasmobranch-balanced salt solution, was administered intravenously (slowly) q 72 hours for five treatments. Twice daily assist feeding of gel food combined with enrofloxacin 10 mg/kg PO q 24 hours for 14 days. The shark began feeding on its own in 2 weeks.

CASE 109

1 What is your diagnostic plan? Fine needle aspirate of the mass and cytology. In this case, a cloudy yellow colored fluid was obtained. Cytology results revealed numerous white blood cells. No bacterial organisms were seen on a Gram stain. A CBC and blood chemistry panel would be helpful in this case.

2 What might be the cause of this condition? The specific cause of the cyst formation is unknown but the presence of numerous white blood cells are indicative of an inflammatory process.

3 How would you manage this case? This superficial localized cyst could resolve spontaneously and require no specific treatment. Initial aspiration or drainage may also be helpful. If the cyst recurs and becomes problematic, the treatment options include surgical removal. The use of systemic antibiotics might be warranted based on blood analysis or evidence of systemic disease.

CASE 110

1 Is there anything in the history that may give a clue to the cause(s) of the current problem?

- Determining the age of the pond can sometimes narrow the list of possible problems. New ponds are more likely to experience 'new tank syndrome' or ammonia toxicity due to immature filtration systems. New ponds are also more likely to have recently introduced fish that can carry pathogens and spread them within the population. However, established ponds undergoing remodeling can also act as 'new ponds' and experience similar problems. Old equipment/filtration systems may have been replaced by new systems and, if the volume has increased, many owners tend to add new fish.

- Automatic feeders are notorious for experiencing failure. Leftover food was observed floating on the pond surface. Purposeful or inadvertent overfeeding can adversely affect water quality.
- Several key components of the life support system are not in use. Water quality problems are likely if there is insufficient filtration (biological and mechanical) and water turnover may be inadequate.
- Water quality evaluation is necessary to complete the minimum database.
- Water testing revealed an ammonia level greater than 8.0 ppm. The pH was 7.8–8.0, which is typical for ponds in the area using the local municipal water supply. Nitrite, nitrate, copper, and hydrogen sulfide levels were all 0. The lack of measurable nitrite and nitrate levels indicates the existing filtration system is inadequate or too immature to handle the current demands.

In addition, the alkalinity (buffering capacity) of the system was extremely low (<10 ppm), making the system susceptible to wide pH fluctuations that can be fatal to the fish. Low alkalinity also adversely affects the biofiltration capacity by reducing the availability of a carbon source, necessary for the health of the nitrifying bacteria.

2 What is your next step? The owner was instructed to remove the automatic feeder, stop feeding temporarily, and perform large water changes based on daily ammonia test results. Alkalinity was temporarily improved with the addition of sodium bicarbonate at each water change based on alkalinity readings. Mesh bags of crushed coral were added to aid in long-term stabilization of the alkalinity levels. Existing filtration equipment was put back online.

With frequent water changes, the increased filtration capacity, routine monitoring of the water quality parameters, and withholding food, the water quality stabilized over the next several weeks. The owner began limited feeding and continued to monitor water quality.

CASE 111

1 What was the likely cause of this wound? The avulsion was apparently caused by a bite from another moray eel in the exhibit. Bite wounds are a common clinical finding in moray exhibits. Minor injury can be left alone for self-recovery but medical intervention may be necessary in severe cases to prevent sepsis.

2 How would you treat these lesions? Surgical correction of an abdominal avulsion was considered in this case. The injured eel was isolated into a tub containing 100 ppm MS-222 immersion for general stage III anesthesia. Due to the long procedure required, a surgical plane of anesthesia was maintained by delivering the aerated anesthetic solution into the buccal cavity using a 1 cm diameter rubber tube connected to a small pump.

The hanging skin flaps were severed using a scalpel. The abdominal cavity was flushed with 200 mL of an abdominal lavage solution (1% enrofloxacin in sterile water) using a sterile feeding tube. The peritoneum was closed using a simple continuous pattern with 3-0 polyglactin suture. The muscular layer was closed using cruciate sutures with 2-0 polyglactin. The wound was flushed with sterile water followed by 5 mL of 1% enrofloxacin. Following the procedure the eel was transferred into anesthetic-free water and recovered from anesthesia within a few minutes.

Enrofloxacin and ketoprofen were administered daily for 3 and 7 days respectively following the surgery. The surgical site was irrigated by sterile saline irrigation, dried by sterile cotton gauze, and then sprayed with 0.01% hypochlorous acid q 48 hours for 10 days. The wound is shown at 7 days post-surgery (**111b**) and was completely healed 3 weeks post-surgery (**111c**).

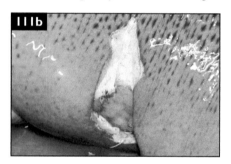 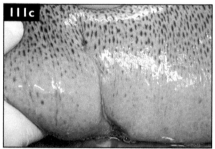

3 How could this condition be prevented? Overcrowding of moray eels may lead to aggressive behaviors. Reducing the population in the exhibit by transferring some individuals to another exhibit or adding more hiding places can help prevent further injuries from aggression brought about by territoriality.

CASE 112

1 What would be your diagnostic plan? Physical examination should be combined with skin scraping of the lesions and blood collection for a CBC and biochemistry. One manta ray was captured for this procedure. The ray was observed to have reddish abrasions, erosions, and ulcerative wounds on its upper and lower jaws, with a severe copepod infection. The cephalic lobes were similarly affected. Furthermore, multifocal clusters of attached copepods accompanied erosions and ulcerative wounds of the right cephalic and posterior area of the right eye area (**112b**). Wet mount microscopic examination of the skin scrape revealed a caligoid copepod (*Lepeophtheirus acutus*) infestation (**112c**) as the cause of the lesions.

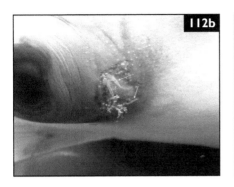

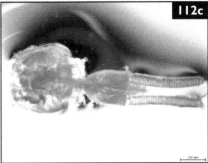

2 How do caligoid copepods affect fish? Caligoid copepods, or sea lice, are crustacean ectoparasites that infest the skin of fish. They scrape the epithelium while feeding and cause physical and enzymatic damage at their sites of attachment, resulting in abrasion-like lesions. Heavy sea lice infestation can cause deep ulcerations and potentially create an entry site for opportunistic pathogens.

3 What is an appropriate treatment strategy? Water-borne administration of organophosphate pesticides (e.g. trichlorfon or dichlorvos) is commonly used to control crustacean ectoparasites in fish. However, these medications carry potential risks not only to elasmobranchs in the exhibit, but also to human health.

Diflubenzuron, a chitin synthesis inhibitor insecticide, is considered an effective and safe treatment at 0.02 mg/L for different species of elasmobranches. Diflubenzuron acts by inhibiting the production of chitin, which is used by caligoid copepods to build the exoskeleton after molting. This results in an incomplete life cycle and ultimate death of the parasite.

With such a large exhibit a number of logistical and financial considerations must be addressed. In this case, the target exposure time was calculated at 8 hours and managed by discontinuing ozonation and foam fractionation during this interval. Food was reduced by 50% for the treatment period, which lasted 3 weeks (q 40 hours for 10 treatments). All the animals fed normally during the treatment period, there were no observable adverse effects, and parasites could not be found after therapy was complete.

CASE 113

1 Are there any other questions you would like to ask? It is important to determine how experienced the owner is with marine systems and further history may reveal a potential traumatic cause for the lesion. Questions would include:

- How long have you been keeping fish?
- How long have you had this fish?

- Are there any other fish/invertebrates in the tank? Any new additions to the tank?
- Is there any life support equipment inside the tank that might cause traumatic or thermal injury?

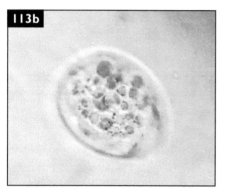

2 What would be your next step? A closer evaluation of the lesion is needed. Wet mount cytology (skin scrape, gill biopsy) and a deep tissue sample for bacterial culture and sensitivity would be the next best steps to complete the minimum database. If the owner allows, a sample for histopathology can also be submitted.

A skin scraping from the margin of the lesions revealed a *Uronema marinum* infestation (**113b**).

The lesion was carefully débrided and silver sulfadiazine 1% ointment applied to the wound. Four weeks of ceftazidime 20 mg/kg IM q 72 hours was dispensed. With each injection, the owner was instructed to apply silver sulfadiazine with a sterile cotton applicator to the wound (**113c**). A 5-day course of metronidazole as an immersion treatment (6.5 mg/L or one crushed 250 mg tablet/10 gals) was chosen to treat the *Uronema*.

The lesion responded well to the treatment regimen and slowly improved (**113d–f**). A piece of necrotic bone was sloughed 1 month after presentation. Ceftazidime was discontinued after 1 month but topical silver sulfadiazine was continued every 3 days for 6 months.

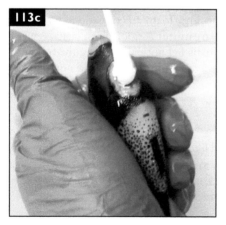

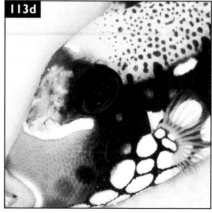

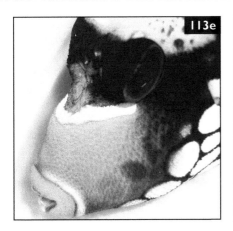 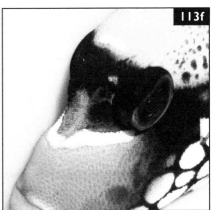

In cases like this, it is important to communicate the possible length of treatment to the owner, and determine if they can administer treatments or will the patient need to be seen by you or your colleagues for treatment. While not used in this fish, a topical misoprostol and phenytoin gel, compounded to order, may speed healing in cases like this.

CASE 114

1 What type of agent is alfaxalone? Alfaxalone is a neurosteroid general anesthetic approved for use in dogs and cats. Like propofol it works by enhancing the gamma-aminobutyric acid receptor.

2 How can it be applied to fish? Alfaxalone is absorbed across the gills and can be used for sedation or general anesthesia. The effects of long-term use are unknown. The effects of IV administration in fish are unknown. Typical induction dose by immersion is approximately 2.5–10 mg/L.

3 Is this compound approved for use in fish intended for human consumption? Alfaxalone is not approved for use in fish and should not be administered to fish in the food chain.

CASE 115

1 What is the cause of these clinical signs? According to recent water quality records, DO levels went up to 114.3% (or 10.57 ppm), consistent with oxygen supersaturation. Cold water naturally holds more oxygen, potentially contributing to gas bubble disease. The air bubbles were most likely absorbed by the branchial vasculature and accumulated in the subcutaneous layers of the octopus.

2 How would you treat this case? The animal had been trained to come to the exhibit's surface. Air aspiration was performed by gently squeezing the affected areas

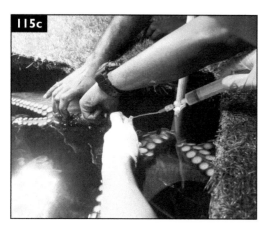

and using a 20G, 2.5 cm (1 in) needle attached to a catheter and three-way valve (**115c**).

3 How can this condition be prevented? Aquarium water becomes dangerous to the aquatic animal when it is oversaturated with gas. Finding the cause of gas supersaturation in the system is essential to prevent similar cases from occurring. Any breaks or leakage in the pipework or pump, which can suck air under pressure and produce excess gas in the water, can potentially lead to a gas supersaturation condition. Close monitoring of DO levels should be done and recorded daily.

CASE 116

1 Based on these findings what should be at the top of your differential list? *Eyrsipelothrix rhusiopathiae* infection. This bacterium is frequently associated with rostral ulceration in freshwater tropical fish.

2 How would you arrive at the diagnosis? Histopathology. Extensive inflammation associated with bacterial colonies between the scales is seen (**116b**, 100×). In a magnified view (**116c**, 400×) of a Brown and Brenn stain (Gram stain) of the area, numerous pleomorphic gram-positive bacteria are observed. This is a zoonotic pathogen so caution should be observed.

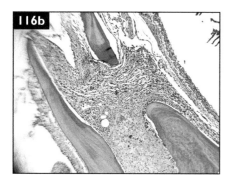

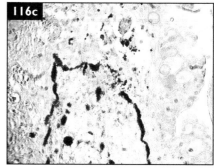

CASE 117

1 What questions would you like to ask the owners? Much more information is needed regarding the system, the fish, and the problem. Some important points to address include:

- What is the water source, is it treated prior to use, and if so, how?
- What is the system set up (number, size and configuration of tanks, filtration equipment, etc.)?
- What are routine management/maintenance procedures (daily, weekly, monthly) including any water changes or addition of drugs, chemicals, or other compounds?
- Are there any survivors in the system prior to addition of new fish, and are they all in the same taxonomic group?

2 What additional diagnostic tests would you recommend? Additional water quality testing based on history, and a more complete work up (including a thorough necropsy, microbiology/culture, and potentially histology). The affected species all prefer soft water, low mineral content, and lower pH. The unaffected species prefer higher pH and salinity. Owing to the problems noted with plant survival, as well as the lack of parasites, the salinity and heavy metals (e.g. copper) should also be checked. In this case, salinity measurements were approximately 7–8 g/L and copper levels were zero. The most likely culprit was hypersalinity. The owners added sodium chloride routinely, forgot to mention it, and had not checked the salt levels recently.

CASE 118

1 Are any of the water quality parameters provided of additional concern in the pet store's system? Yes, pH and alkalinity seem a bit low for a pet store system. Although many of the affected species prefer a lower pH in the wild, these species, and especially their domesticated counterparts, have the ability to acclimate to a higher pH. The low pH and alkalinity could indicate chronic loss of buffering capacity, which may lead to a pH crash.

2 What additional water quality data would be necessary for a more complete picture of the system? Source water parameters should always be evaluated – after it has been allowed to aerate for a few hours in a bucket or other inert container – for any case. This allows for a more accurate assessment of the progression of specific parameters, as well as verification of management protocols (water changes, addition of other compounds e.g. salt). If the source water (after aeration) had the following values: total ammonia nitrogen 0, nitrite 0, pH 7.8, temperature 25°C (77°F), DO 7 mg/L, alkalinity 170 mg/L $CaCO_3$, hardness 170 mg/L $CaCO_3$, salinity 0, then it would be clear that the tank pH and alkalinity have in fact progressed downward (vs. if the source water had a pH of 6.8 and alkalinity of 51 mg/L, which would indicate most likely a high water exchange rate), and that salt had been added to the system.

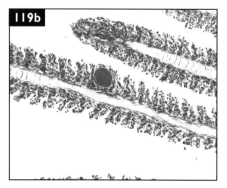

CASE 119

1 What is the cause of these lesions and how would you treat this condition? The structures (the blue object on H&E, **119b**) are epitheliocystis, caused by infection with Chlamydiales bacteria. Chlamydiales is an order of obligate intracellular bacteria that primarily affect gills, although they can occasionally be found in other organs. These infections often respond to immersion treatment with oxytetracycline.

CASE 120

1 What are these structures? These structures are myxozoan spores (each with two polar capsules). This species is most likely *Myxobolus balantiocheili*. *M. balantiocheili* has been reported in the literature, and apparently causes damage and clinical signs via compression and degeneration of the CNS around the large cysts, with minimal inflammation.

2 What would you recommend to the wholesaler? Depopulation, even though there may be low probability of spread in a closed system. There are currently no established or effective chemotherapeutics available for treatment of myxozoa in fish. The complex life cycle of other *Myxobolus* spp. suggests that an invertebrate intermediate host (possibly an oligochaete worm) is likely required for completion of the life cycle.

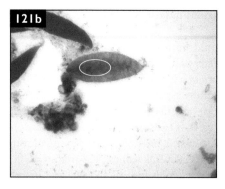

CASE 121

1 What are these organisms? *Protoopalina symphysodonis*, an opalinid occasionally seen concurrent with *Spironucleus vortens* in the intestines of gourami and discus. A Diff-Quik® stain (**121b**) reveals the presence of two nuclei.

2 Do you recommend treating for this condition? It is considered to be an endocommensal organism and no specific treatment is required.

CASE 122

1 How would you approach this case? Once you have taken a complete history and examined the fish in the transport container, sedation and skin and gill biopsies are warranted. You do this and the tissue samples look normal under the microscope. In addition, since the owner does not report nitrate levels, you should test the water sample for this nitrogenous waste compound. You obtain a reading of 250 mg/L.

2 What recommendations will you have for this client? The most likely problem is nitrate toxicity due to build up of nitrate in the aquarium. Without regular water changes and live plants to assimilate nitrate, these levels are consistent with the history. While nitrate is the least toxic of the major nitrogen compounds in a biological system, it has been determined that some species are more sensitive to nitrate than others. Clinical signs can include unthriftiness, goiter in elasmobranchs, and even death in certain species of sturgeon.

CASE 123

1 What are they and what is the likely cause? The structures are granulomas, which are caused by the kinetoplastid flagellate *Cryptobia iubilans*. Approximately 100× magnification is used to view the granulomas. It primarily affects the stomach and upper intestine of African cichlids and discus. Granulomas are formed by the fish in response to the parasite (**123b, c**). In heavy infections, the parasite can disseminate to affect other organs in the coelom. Often the organisms are not observed on wet mounts of the stomach and upper intestine, despite an intense granulomatous response.

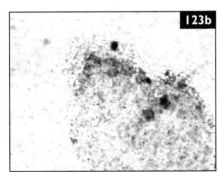 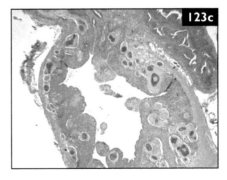

2 How would you manage this problem? The parasite is difficult to eliminate, and management should include water quality improvement, reduction in stocking density, and high quality nutrition. There are several options for oral treatment; 20 mg metronidazole per g of feed or 4.4 mg 2-amino-5-nitrothiazol per g of feed. Both are fed at 1.5% of body weight twice daily for 5–7 days. Affected discus often have concurrent *Spironucleus* infestations.

Answers

CASE 124

1 What is this tissue (most likely) and what are the primary lesions seen in 124a, b? Posterior kidney (**124a**, tubules) and spleen (**124b**). The primary lesions are granulomas (encapsulated structures), not to be confused with the pigmented macrophage aggregates that are not encapsulated.

2 Bench top stains and histology were negative for acid-fast bacteria. What might explain this? What other bacterial disease should be high on the differential list and what additional diagnostics would be required? Acid-fast bacteria (AFB) negative results could be due to differences in staining protocols or because the disease is not caused by *Mycobacterium*. Laboratories differ in the type of acid-fast protocol used and this may affect intensity of staining and observation of the organisms. Some of the various protocols include Ziehl-Neelsen, Kinyoun, and Fite's, and differences occur in the use of acid alcohol or sulfuric acid during the procedure. For suspect mycobacterial cases that are AFB negative on histology, check with the laboratory and consider other AFB protocols.

Franciselliosis was diagnosed in this case, based on growth on modified Thayer Martin media (*Francisella* does not grow on blood agar) and PCR identification, from both culture and tissues.

Franciselliosis is an important emerging disease of fish, first identified in tilapia, but now seen in other species, including hybrid striped bass, fairy wrasses, and damselfish. *Francisella* should be considered as a differential in cases of chronic mortalities with primary findings of splenic and renal granulomas that are AFB negative.

CASE 125

1 What would your recommendation be to this public aquarium? Franciselliosis in warm water species (including tilapia) is often correlated with water quality issues, including cooler temperatures. Depending on the severity of the outbreak and eventual disposition of the fish, depopulation may be a good option to prevent spread of the disease. Studies on the epidemiology and use of various management techniques to reduce morbidity and mortality are ongoing, but more is needed. Culture and sensitivity should be run to identify the best antibiotic (and, for food fish, legalities must be observed), but oxytetracycline has demonstrated some effectiveness, especially if the disease is identified early. Increasing temperatures gradually to 30°C (86°F) may also help reduce mortalities. After quarantine (or depopulation), all tanks, filters, equipment, and supplies used should be properly disinfected prior to re-use.

CASE 126

1 What are these structures? Axillary glands, which are common to catfish, and the source of the venom that can cause pain when skin is punctured by one of their fin spines. Rubbing the punctured area with the mucus of the catfish will quickly alleviate pain.

CASE 127

1 What are these structures? Pentastomid nymphs. Pentastomids, although worm-like in appearance, are actually crustacean parasites with an indirect life cycle. This species is most likely *Sebekia mississippiensis*, where fish are the intermediate hosts and the final hosts are aquatic reptiles including alligators, aquatic snakes, and aquatic turtles. Adult pentastomids inhabit the respiratory tract of these animals.

2 What management options would you recommend to the producer? Production of live-bearers (including swordtail, platies, and guppies) in Florida often includes stocking of newly cleaned ponds with male and female broodstock, but allowing fish continued reproduction over the course of several years. If ponds are not cleaned out and re-worked at least once a year, they can be colonized by aquatic reptiles, thereby perpetuating the life cycle for this parasite. Recommendations would be more frequent pond cleaning, removal and/or methods to reduce invasion by aquatic reptiles, and routine surveillance for these hosts and of the fish for infection. Although some species of fish often show no behavioral signs and continue to eat, other species may experience significant morbidity and mortality. In this case, the fish did not experience mortalities, behaved normally, but were not sellable. As there is no way to treat or manage this condition, euthanasia is recommended.

CASE 128

1 What additional information do you need? Additional information (this list is not comprehensive) would include:
- Were there any previous problems with fish from these suppliers?
- Did any bags of koi in these shipments arrive and remain normal?
- Determine system water quality: total ammonia nitrogen, nitrite, DO, pH, temperature, alkalinity, hardness, carbon dioxide, salinity.
- Determine the differences in arrival bag water quality (including temperature) vs. the system water quality.
- Were anesthetics used in shipping?

Answers

2 What are some differential diagnoses and how would you rule these out?

- Water quality issues: differences, for example in pH and temperature, could cause significant stress on the fish. Inadequate degassing in the system, leading to build of carbon dioxide, could cause problems. A chemical treatment (e.g. formalin, copper) added to the water might have been enough to further compromise these fish.

- Shipping problem: history or observation for oxygenation problems (flat bags, flight delays), anesthetic overdose?

- Infectious disease: rule out viral, bacterial, fungal, and parasitic etiologies via biopsy, necropsy, blood analysis. The temperatures are compatible with carp edema virus (CEV, also termed koi sleepy disease), caused by a poxvirus. This would be high on the differential list given the unusual behavior of the affected koi. Other clinical signs that support this diagnosis include hemorrhage, pale swollen gills, enophthalmia, and mortalities. CEV has been identified worldwide, and histology and PCR would confirm this etiology. Although addition of sodium chloride (5 g/L) may help reduce morbidity and mortality, such information is anecdotal. Depopulation should be considered. This specific case was confirmed as CEV. Koi herpesvirus should be considered, especially if the gill pathology included necrotic areas (red/white) gills, and could be ruled out using culture and/or PCR of affected tissues. Temperatures are too warm for spring viremia of carp (SVC), but information on the exporting facility water temperatures and a disease history would be helpful.

CASE 129

1 Which koi is abnormal, and why? The bottom koi is abnormal. The most pronounced deformity is the anteriorly to posteriorly flattened skull/face. It also has an abnormal caudal peduncle that appears thin and shortened.

2 Given the history, what are some probable causes for this abnormality and what would be your management recommendations? Although there are a number of non-infectious and infectious possible causes, high on the differential list should be a nutritional deficiency or imbalance. Vitamin C deficiency is most commonly associated with skeletal deformities in fish but development of stabilized forms, and better storage procedures, have helped reduce deformities in general. The history should address feed expiration dates, method of storage, and examination of the label. Specific nutrient testing might be required. Since cyprinids are agastric, the most critical historical information is the tilapia diet. Fish meal (which includes a significant portion of bone) is a common source of calcium and phosphorus for fish with true stomachs (which allow for acid digestion and breakdown into constituent ions). Fish can absorb calcium from the water for their requirements, and since the pond water had moderate hardness, it is likely that calcium is less of

an issue than phosphorus. Koi and other cyprinids must have a diet that includes inorganic forms of phosphate (e.g. calcium monobasic phosphate) that are more bioavailable. The producer should switch feed to a carp/koi specific diet with the appropriate form of phosphorus. Of course, a more thorough necropsy/work up should be undertaken to rule out other factors.

CASE 130

1 What are these protists? *Ichthyobodo,* kinetoplastid flagellates (**130b**, arrows), are attached to the epithelium of the skin in this histologic photomicrograph. *Ichthyobodo* infestations are extremely irritating to fish, which respond to the presence of the parasite by producing excess mucus. The abundant mucus is the source of the gray sheen of affected fish.

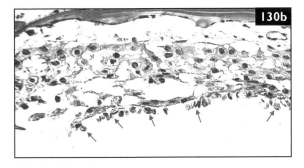

2 How would you treat this condition? These small flagellates can be difficult to control because the excess mucus can shield them from chemotherapeutics. Multiple treatments with formalin may be necessary.

CASE 131

1 What recommendations can you make with regard to the following parameters?

Food. Do not feed fish during a power outage. In warmer months eating and digesting will use valuable oxygen. In winter fish will likely have plenty of oxygen but because of their slowed metabolism they will probably be uninterested in food. Furthermore, uneaten food will only pollute the aquarium or pond with unnecessary nitrogen.

Temperature. In winter, try and insulate the aquarium with a blanket, sleeping bag, or newspapers. In summer, remove anything from the surface of the water in an effort to increase the surface area and hence gas exchange efficiency. Obtain an aquarium thermometer and have it handy to monitor the water temperature. Most tropical fish can tolerate temperatures of around 16°C (61°F) for several hours.

Answers

Once temperatures dip to <14°C (<57°F) action should be taken to elevate the temperature. Here are some options:

- Obtain an alternate power supply to run the heater and pump/filter. This could be a generator or creatively used extension cord to a location with power.
- Obtain an alternate and safe external heat source such as a propane or kerosene heater.
- Physically transport the fish to a warmer location. Heavy-duty zip-lock bags work well for this purpose. Fill the bag with one-third water and two-thirds air. Pure oxygen is even better than air. As long as the external temperature is adequate, sparsely packed fish (2 cm of fish per liter; 5 inches of fish per US gallon) should survive for at least 36 hours packed in this manner. Alternatively, any secure vessel such as a bucket, tub, or large jar can be used to move fish to a safe location. While moving the entire aquarium is an option, it will usually present some logistical challenges. If one decides to move the aquarium, then up to 70% of the water may be discarded before the move to make transport easier (remember, 1 L of water weighs 1 kg, and 1 US gal of water weighs 8 lb).
- If the problem is water that gets too warm, then make sure exposure to direct sunlight is minimized or eliminated completely. In most situations tropical and even temperate fish, like goldfish and koi, should be able to tolerate water temperatures of 30°C (86°F) or even 32°C (90°F) for a day or more. One risk of prolonged exposure to these high temperatures is low DO. Manually stirring the water with a whisk or similar implement can help elevate oxygen levels until power returns.
- In the case that the fish cannot be moved, and the water temperature reaches a critically low level, warm dechlorinated water can be added to the aquarium. A thermometer should be used to be certain that acute changes do not exceed 2°C (5°F). Generally, a 10% water change with warm water every hour or two should safely increase an aquarium's temperature without endangering the fish.
- Temperate species such as goldfish and koi should be fine without changing anything in the environment. If the power outage persists and the surface of a pond freezes over, the ice can be mechanically broken to form an 'air hole.'
- Only as an absolute last resort should fish from one aquarium or pond be mixed with fish from another aquatic system. This practice greatly increases the risk of spreading infectious viral, bacterial, fungal, and parasitic diseases. It may also lead to inter- or intra-specific aggression.

Water quality. The longer fish remain in unfiltered water the worse water quality parameters will become. Most fish can survive days or even weeks without food. If ammonia levels increase above 1.0 ppm, then water changes (10–30%) are recommended.

Lighting. The least of your worries. Ornamental fish will survive indefinitely without fluorescent/supplemental lighting. This is of more concern with tropical reef aquaria where live sponges and coral are maintained. Many of these invertebrate species rely on bright light and the symbiotic organisms the light supports.

CASE 132

1 How can you account for these results? Nearly 6 months without water changes have likely allowed for the build up of organic acids and other waste products to the point where the pH has dropped to a dangerous level. The elevated ammonia is likely due to the compromised biofilter; nitrifying bacteria do not function well in acid water, especially below a pH of 5.5. The water is also a poor buffer (relatively low alkalinity) so this compounds the problem of pH stabilization.

2 What are your recommendations? Slow, gradual water changes over the next week to 10 days. A reasonable recommendation would be 20% per day until the pH stabilizes at a healthy level (7.5–8.0 for tilapia). Recommend that the owner returns to their regular water change practices and test the water at least once a month.

CASE 133

1 What items would you include on such a list? (1) A net (note: herding fish into a plastic bag using a net is safer than using a net on its own; nets can damage the protective mucus layer and sensitive epidermis); (2) bucket(s); (3) dechlorinating agent; (4) phone number for your fish veterinarian; (5) phone number of the nearest pet store; (6) propane or kerosene heater; (7) rubber bands (to close bags in case zip-lock bags are unavailable); (8) salt (aquarium, kosher); (9) spare aquarium heater; (10) thermometer(s); (11) water testing kit; (12) zip-lock bags (various sizes).

CASE 134

1 What questions would you like to ask the owners? Some further history would be helpful as you assemble your diagnostic and potential therapy plans. This list includes most of the pertinent topics but is not comprehensive:
- Is the fish eating? If so, how much and how frequently?
- How big is the pond?
- Are there other fish in the pond?
- Are any of these fish showing clinical/similar signs?
- Were there any electrical storms about the time you noticed the problem?

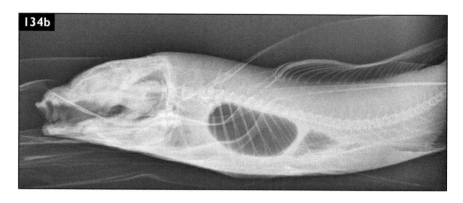

134b

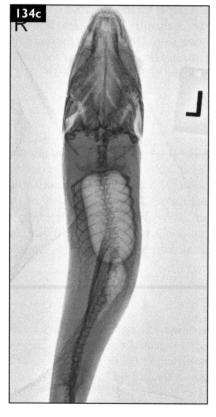

134c R

2 **What diagnostic tests would you recommend?** You learn that the koi is eating but must be hand fed. The owners are very committed to their fish and agree to have the fish imaged with radiography and ultrasonography. Computed tomography was recommended but the owners declined due to cost and the fact that the imaging performed (**134b, c**) revealed an abnormal swim bladder (enlarged cranial segment and small caudal segment), tail curvature, and normal appearing vertebral column. Other diagnostic tests would include water quality evaluation, skin and gill biopsies, and possibly blood work.

With no history of an electrical storm or power surge, nor having any other fish affected and good water quality in the pond, a decision was made to empirically treat the koi with antibiotics (enrofloxacin, 10 mg/kg ICe q 96 hours for four treatments) and 1.2 ppt salt in the hospital tank (1 pound salt/100 US gal).

The koi gradually improved and within 1 month was completely normal according to the owners and back in the main pond (**134d,** the fish 1 year after treatment). Three years later the koi is hungry, active, and behaving normally. This positive outcome cannot be definitively linked

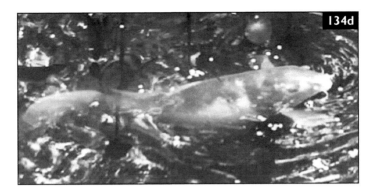

to the treatment. It is possible, if not likely, that supportive care and nutritional support contributed greatly to the case management success.

CASE 135

1 Why was the question about electrical storms included with the history taking? Lightning strikes close to koi ponds have been linked to spinal luxations and subsequent scoliosis in affected fish. When such an event occurs not all fish in the pond are injured and, in fact, frequently just one or two animals are involved. Electrical power surges from faulty pumps or other electrical fixtures/wires can also result in spinal deformity and musculoskeletal disease.

CASE 136

1 What concerns do you have when handling electric eels? Electric eels have specialized electric organs capable of discharging low-amperage bursts of electricity. These organs are serially connected and electric surges can exceed 600 volts depending on the length of the

fish, with the highest voltage measured at the head and tail. Special handling protocols and equipment must be used to ensure patient and staff safety. To avoid inadvertent electric shocks, personnel involved with handling of the fish should wear rubber boots and thick, rubberized gloves (**136b**). Additionally, it is

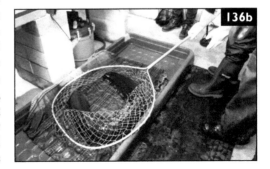

useful if equipment such as transport containers, nets, and restraint devices are made out of non-conductive materials.

2 **What diagnostic tests would you recommend?**

* Anesthesia is required for proper examination of the affected area.
* Radiography can be used to assess how long the nail is, if the nail is intact,

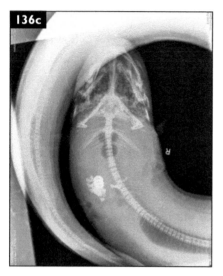

and if other foreign material is present. Radiography can also give information about the extent of the soft tissue trauma caused by the nail. A dorsoventral radiography image taken of the cranial part of the electric eel after the nail was removed showed two metal washers and some small stones in the stomach (**136c**).

* In the absence of imaging technology a metal detector may be used to see if metal can be found.

3 **How would you perform anesthesia in this case? How would you assess depth of anesthesia during induction?** The animal was anesthetized in a separate induction tank containing 300 mg/L tricaine methanesulphonate (MS-222) in dechlorinated municipal water with an equal amount of sodium bicarbonate as a buffer. After 20 minutes, the fish was sedate and a proper examination of the affected area could be performed. After pulling out the screw, GI content exited through the perforated wound in the body wall. A stomach perforation was suspected and it was decided to perform an exploratory celiotomy. As depth of anesthesia was not adequate to perform surgery, 0.11 mg/kg medetomidine and 2.2 mg/kg ketamine were administered intramuscularly (IM). Once a surgical plane of anesthesia was reached, the fish was taken out of the water and placed on a plastic table for surgery. Aerated water containing MS-222 from the induction tank was circulated over the gills every 2–5 minutes throughout the procedure using a 60 mL syringe. At the end of the procedure 0.28 mg/kg atipamezole was given IM to reverse the effects of the medetomidine. Once the eel was fully recovered it was returned to its aquarium.

To evaluate depth of anesthesia during induction, the response to stimuli and ability to right itself were evaluated. A voltmeter with the electrodes placed in the water, cranially at the head and caudally near the tail, was used to detect if the eel was still discharging. As voltage discharges by electric eels are voluntarily controlled, the discharges can be used to assess depth of anesthesia. As depth of anesthesia increased, less current could be measured and during surgery, no current was detected. A Doppler was used to measure and monitor heart rate.

CASE 137

1 What is this organism? Egg of a capsalid monogenean.

2 Would you recommend treatment and if so, with what? Even though adults may not be observed, treatment is recommended. Praziquantel is the drug of choice, and can be used as a prolonged immersion at 5 mg/L for 3 weeks.

CASE 138

1 What is this structure? It is an egg of an ancyrocephalid monogenean that is the most common monogenean gill parasite of non-cyprinids. The eggs are impervious to treatment, so treatment must be applied several times to control the parasite. Praziquantel is the drug of choice and is applied at 5 mg/L for 3 weeks.

CASE 139

1 Provide a summary of SVCv. This highly infectious disease is caused by *Rhabdovirus carpio*. It is global in nature and affects fish of the family Cyprinidae; some examples include goldfish (*Carassius auratus*), carp/koi (*Cyprinus carpio*), golden orfe (*Leuciscus idus*), and tench (*Tinca tinca*). Clinical signs can include abdominal distension, skin and branchial hemorrhage, exophthalmia, pale gills, and distension/protrusion of the vent (**139a, b**). Early in the course of disease, affected fish may appear weak and congregate in areas of still water.

2 What are your obligations as a licensed USDA APHIS accredited veterinarian when dealing with a suspected case? All suspect cases should be necropsied and the US Department of Agriculture (USDA) contacted for proper diagnostic sample routing. Confirmed cases must be reported to the USDA and state veterinarian.

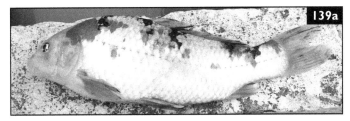

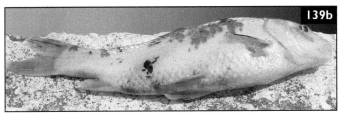

Answers

3 How would you proceed to collect and submit samples? A minimum of 10 moribund fish or 10 fish exhibiting clinical signs should be collected and sent live to the laboratory or killed and packed separately in sealed aseptic containers on ice. Depending on the size of fish, whole fish (body length between 0 and 4 cm) or the entire viscera including kidney and encephalon (body length is between 4 and 6 cm) should be collected. If the fish is larger, liver, kidney, spleen, and encephalon should be collected aseptically. Samples should be combined to form pools of a maximum of five fish per pool (each pool should not weigh more than 1.5 g). Tissues should be placed in sterile vials and stored at 4°C (39.2°F) until virus extraction is performed at the laboratory (the OIE [World Animal Health Organization] recommends testing begins within 24 hours of sample collection). For detecting asymptomatic carriers, tissue samples of kidney, spleen, gill, and encephalon should be collected. Depending on the population size, fish collection must encompass a statistically significant number of specimens. The sampling should be designed to enable detection, at a 95% confidence level, of infected animals.

4 What type of legal follow-up is required for affected facilities? Facilities testing positive have to follow the recommendations described in the International Aquatic Animal Health Code and the Diagnostic Manual for Aquatic Animal Diseases by OIE to be declared free of SVCv. In the USA, the USDA recommendations would need to be adhered to.

CASE 140

1 What are your next steps? Test the water. You do this and find the temperature, pH, ammonia, nitrite, nitrate, total alkalinity, and DO are within normal limits.

Examine the moribund fish and obtain gill, skin, and fin biopsy samples. You complete these tasks and do not observe any pathogens; however, there appears to be excess mucus associated with the gill lamellae (**140b**).

Review the history with the owner and expand on it if possible. Based on your experience and the current test results you suspect a toxic event, perhaps from a

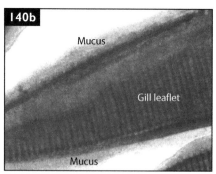

heavy metal. When queried about the possibility of any copper piping being associated with the plumbing, the owner mentions that copper is being used as an algicide and parasiticide in the pond. Further discussion reveals the presence of a commercially available copper ion exchanger (that had been turned off 3 days prior). The owner reports maintaining total copper levels below 0.2 ppm using test strips provided by the company. Well water (the pond's water source), used as a control, tested zero using the owner's test strips (**140c**). The pond water, despite a 30% water change the previous day, registered between 0.05 and 0.1 ppm copper (**140d**).

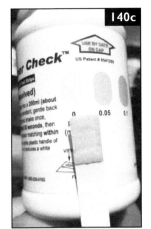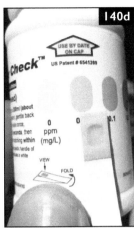

You have the owner disconnect the ion exchanger, add activated carbon to the system, institute daily 20–30% water changes, and add 1.5 ppt salt to the pond. In addition, you send water samples to a toxicology laboratory for further testing. The analysis finds 0.123 ppm copper in the pond water. Following disconnection of the ion exchanger no further problems were noted with the fish.

CASE 141

1 What diagnostic procedures can be performed to diagnose the cause of coelomic distension? Coelomic ultrasonography images were difficult to interpret due to the small size of the individual. Some irregular shadowing was present, but no pocket of fluid distension was noted. Radiographs showed a large accumulation of gravel within the GI tract, due to substrate ingestion within the exhibit (**141b**). Fine needle aspiration should be

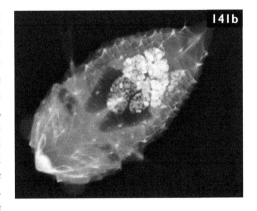

considered in similar cases, but due to lack of visible distension or swelling during examination, there was no effective target to aspirate.

2 What considerations in the exhibit and husbandry might be taken to reduce the incidence of this condition? Some fish species or individuals are prone to substrate ingestion, and the size of loose substrate should be considered in relation to the size of inhabitants and potential for obstruction if consumed. Excessive food

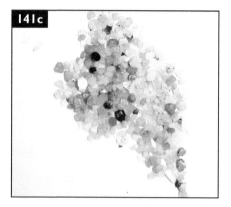

competition and/or feeding excessively to allow food to fall to the bottom may contribute to fish foraging off the substrate and accidental ingestion. This fish was removed from the exhibit into a tank without substrate and it passed a large amount of gravel (**141c**). After a second episode of gravel ingestion, it was subsequently released into the wild, where it had been collected.

CASE 142

1 How could you further pursue diagnostics in this case? Histopathology. In this case, severe coccidial disease was diagnosed on histopathology (**142c**). The coccidial organisms can be observed in the intestinal villi at both 200× (**142c**, arrows) and 600× (**142d**, arrows) magnifications. The structures seen on the wet mounts could be inflammatory cells, coccidia, or a combination of both.

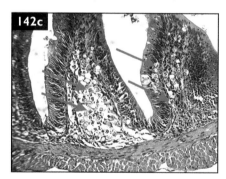
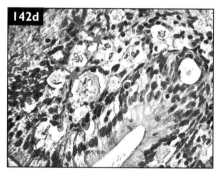

CASE 143

1 What measurements should your receptionist request from the client in order to accurately determine the volume and what equation would you use? If one knows the length, height, and width of a rectangular or square aquarium, volume can be calculated by multiplying these three values (in centimeters or inches) to give either cubic centimeters or cubic inches. To determine liters divide the total by 1,000, and to determine US gallons divide the total by 231 (cubic inches/US gallon). For example, in this case, the client's aquarium measures 183 cm (72 in) long,

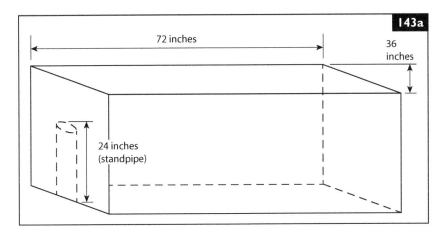

91.5 cm (36 in) wide, and 61 cm (24 in) high. This comes to 1,021 L or 270 US gal. For accuracy, when it comes to determining water volume the values for calculation should be for the water dimensions and not total tank measurements (**143a**).

2 If this were a cylindrical aquarium, what measurements would you need and in what equation? For cylinders one needs to know the radius and depth to calculate volume. The formula is: $\pi r^2 \times$ height = volume. Pi (π) equals 3.142, r is the radius of the cylinder, and height the vertical measurement of water (**143b**).

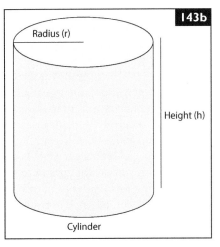

CASE 144

1 What is the likely cause of the problem? Spores of microsporidia are observed in the wet mount of muscle tissue. Histology confirms extensive infection with microsporidia, a fungal parasite that commonly infects danios, and demonstrates the infiltration and destruction of the muscles (**144c, d,** 400×). If an acid-fast stain is performed,

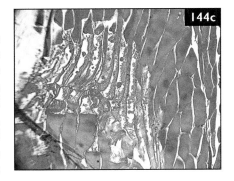

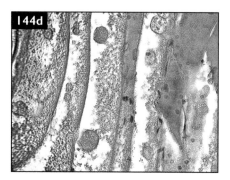

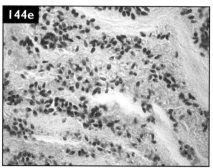

some of the spores would be acid-fast positive (**144e**). There is no treatment for microsporidiosis, and it is directly infective to other fish in the tank. Any affected fish should be promptly removed and euthanized.

CASE 145

1 What is your diagnostic plan? You thoroughly examine the exhibit and note there are a number of coins on the bottom. The curator, in an exasperated tone, says that despite the large signs warning people not to throw anything into the exhibit, visitors continue to toss coins into the water. The aquarist responsible for the exhibit removes the coins every Sunday morning and they use the money to buy fish food about twice a year.

You decide to anesthetize and closely examine the two affected trout. While you are doing this you ask the curator to begin thawing the frozen trout in warm water. Gill, skin, and fin biopsies of the moribund trout are all negative but the gills look pale. You draw blood samples from the caudal hemal arch and using the centrifuge in the museum's small veterinary laboratory you determine that one fish has a packed cell volume (PCV) of 8% and the other a PCV of 5%.

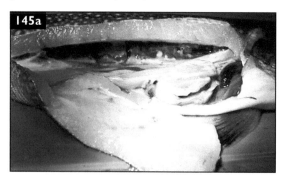

Next, you necropsy the thawed trout, and immediately note how pale the musculature is (**145a**). Further along you explore the stomach and find a 1995 US penny that is mildly corroded (**145b**). All US pennies made after 1983 are 96% zinc. Elevated zinc levels are known to cause anemia in many species. The liver was subsequently analyzed and found to have 833 ppm zinc. While there are no reference ranges for zinc in salmonids, this appears to be a very high number compared with other published studies.

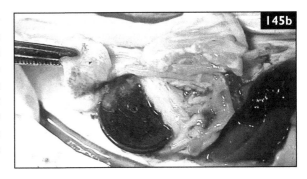

2 What are your recommendations? You recommend radiographing the moribund trout to rule out GI foreign bodies. If coins or other foreign objects are identified, options to remove these items should be pursued (non-surgical and surgical).

CASE 146

1 What additional history questions are important in this case? Additional history is very important in a case like this, as there are many possible causes of cataracts in fish (nutritional deficiencies, excessive UV light exposure, parasites, genetics, trauma, osmotic and temperature changes, toxins, etc.). Additional history for the individual fish is also important, as this may affect diagnostic and treatment recommendations. The following questions cover important topics, although additional information could also be collected as part of a complete history:

- Describe the tank set-up, filtration systems, water change protocols, water quality testing, and feeding type/frequency. Have there been any changes in feed recently?
- What is the source of this animal and how long has it been maintained in the collection? Have there been recent additions to the tank?
- Is this animal housed singly? If not, what other kinds of animals are in the tank and how many are there?
- Are any of the other animals in the tank affected?
- Has this animal showed any difficulty eating or navigating the exhibit?
- Is there any history of trauma? Has there been progression of the disease since it was first noted? Have any treatments been attempted, and if so, what were the results?

In this case, the animal was a wild-caught long-term member of a stable tank system. The tank was stocked with an appropriate number of similarly-sized conspecifics, and husbandry was adequate. No trauma was observed prior to development of the cataract. The cataract appeared stable since it was first noticed, and no treatments had been attempted. The fish was eating well and navigating appropriately.

Answers

2 What diagnostic tests are indicated? Baseline diagnostics, such as a skin scrape, gill clip, and blood work, are never wrong in a case like this; however, these tests are unlikely to shed light on the cause of the cataract or aid in cataract management. Specific diagnostics to consider for an animal with a cataract include an electroretinogram (ERG). If the retina is no longer functional, recommendations for management of this cataract may change.

In this case, an ERG was not pursued because the animal was clinically doing well. Since this was a display animal, the cataract was being addressed for cosmetic reasons and due to long-term concern for the health of the eye secondary to progression of the cataract. Note: ERG evaluations have been successfully performed in fish, and should be pursued in any case where vision is important.

3 What management options will you propose for this animal? As in other species, cataracts in fish are managed surgically. Surgical options include phacoemulsification, phakectomy, and enucleation. If this were a pet fish, continued monitoring of the cataract could also be considered.

CASE 147

1 How would you manage this challenge? Manual extraction (phakectomy) was required. This was not unexpected due to the density of fish lenses. However, phacoemulsification is recommended over phakectomy due to the sheer size of the fish lens, the inability of their iris to dilate, and the decreased risk of damage to the posterior lens capsule. Consultation with a veterinary ophthalmologist is highly recommended for cataract management in fish (**147a** shows the eye being prepared for surgery).

2 How would you manage this case after surgery? Post-operatively, this animal was managed with two injections of a non-steroidal anti-inflammatory pain medication (ketoprofen, 2mg/kg IM q 24 hours). No major post-operative complications were encountered and the fish's appearance was much improved (**147b**).

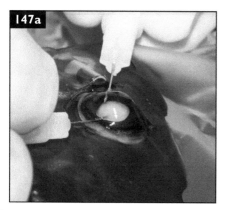

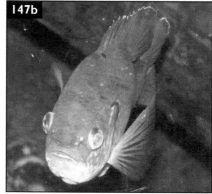

CASE 148

1 Name the cells indicated by the letters and arrows. A, thrombocyte; B, erythrocyte; C, heterophil (leukocyte).

CASE 149

1 What immediately strikes you as abnormal about the *in-situ* visceral cavity? The visceral cavity is filled with a large white mass of what appears to be adipose tissue.

2 How can you quickly confirm the constitution of the large white mass? Confirmation could be made by testing to see if the tissue (a small piece) floats in water or formalin.

3 What may have led to this condition? This is likely the result of a captive diet not consistent with what this New World cichlid eats in the wild. The fish had been fed almost exclusively cichlid pellets. While such commercial diets are an important part of a captive diet, they are almost certainly not representative of the animal's natural food sources. It is recommended that hobbyists learn as much as they can about the fish they are keeping and then work to build an appropriate nutritional plan. In addition to the excessive amount of abdominal fat, this fish also had an idiopathic polycystic liver (visible just below the adipose tissue). Histopathology confirmed this was neither an infectious nor a neoplastic condition.

CASE 150

1 What do you suspect and how will you confirm your suspicion? Histopathology of the affected eyes reveals numerous metacercariae, an encysted stage of digenean trematodes. The results (**150c, d**) demonstrate the presence of many metacercariae in the lens of one of the affected fish. It is unlikely that treatment will be effective, given the location. Although the condition is cosmetically unappealing, it is limited to one eye, and the affected fish may live an otherwise normal life.

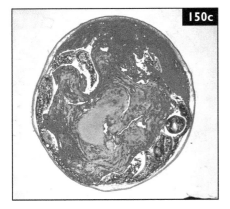
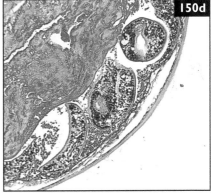

Answers

CASE 151

1 What do you suspect? *Spironucleus vortens*, a diplomonad parasite, is the most likely culprit. On wet mounts, it can be easily confused with *Cryptobia iubilans*, but the latter has not been observed in angelfish. *Spironucleus* primarily inhabits the lower intestinal tract, whereas *C. iubilans* primarily resides in the stomach and upper intestine. Treatment for *Spironucleus* is metronidazole-medicated feed (100 mg/kg body weight for 3 days), or a metronidazole bath for anorexic fish (25 mg/L every other day for three treatments). The environment and diet should be examined to be sure they are appropriate; stressors can exacerbate *Spironucleus* infestations. A scanning electron micrograph shows a *Spironucleus* organism from the intestine of a *Trichogaster* gourami (**151c**).

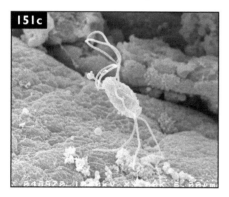

CASE 152

1 What is this condition? Columnaris disease, caused by *Flavobacterium columnare*. Some fish species appear to be more susceptible to columnaris, especially after handling or transport. Many catfishes are susceptible. It may present as the primary infection but can be complicated with secondary opportunistic bacterial infections.

2 What treatment do you recommend? After water quality parameters are analyzed to ensure they are adequate, treatment should consist of the following: increase salinity to 3 ppt or higher if the affected fish will tolerate it; feed a medicated feed containing oxytetracycline; perform a bath with oxytetracycline. Specialized media, such as Cytophaga or Shieh, are often necessary to culture this bacterium.

CASE 153

1 What further diagnostics should be performed? Further diagnostics should include sterile culture of the brain and head kidney for bacteriology and subsequent antibiotic sensitivity and histopathology. Identification of the bacterial growth can be made using traditional microbiological methods utilizing a combination of staining characteristics, cell morphology, and biochemical and physiologic tests. Pure culture isolates can be screened via PCR.

2 What is the diagnosis? Diagnostics reveal a gram-negative rod that is a facultative anaerobe and weakly motile by peritrichous flagella. It is oxidase negative and fermentative in glucose motility deeps (GMD). A reaction of K/A and H_2S negative is produced utilizing triple sugar iron slants. Additionally, it is indole and citrate negative. The API 20E system produces a code of 4204000 that identifies the bacterial growth as *Edwardsiella ictaluri*. *E. ictaluri* is confirmed by PCR and further identifies this to be a danio strain different from the channel catfish strain. Histopathology reveals a severe multifocally extensive to diffuse, systemic disease consistent with *E. ictaluri* infection, characterized by tissue necrosis and large numbers of bacteria often within macrophages in the kidney, spleen, liver, nares, brain, and endomeninges.

CASE 154

1 Identify this parasite (154a) that was found in the small intestine of a fish on the necropsy floor. This is a cestode, distinguishable by the scolex (head/attachment area) and numerous proglottids (reproductive segments).

2 How does this parasite feed? Briefly discuss its life cycle. This parasite feeds by attaching to the GI mucosa and then absorbing nutrients directly from the host gut (cestodes lack their own GI tract). A number of cestodes can be seen attached to the GI mucosa (**154b**). As the cestode grows it develops multiple egg packets called proglottids that are passed in the feces. Once they reach the environment they are consumed by an invertebrate, such as a crustacean, which is then consumed by a fish, the definitive host. In mammals, birds, and reptiles the life cycle is frequently more complicated with multiple intermediate hosts and parasitic life stages.

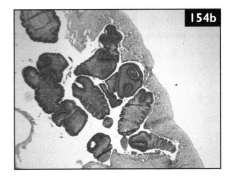

3 If you were to treat this condition, how would you accomplish this? Praziquantel, either by immersion or parenterally, is the drug of choice for cestode management. In some cases the worms will be expelled alive and intact (**154c, d**).

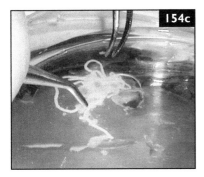
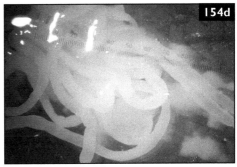

CASE 155

1 What lesion(s) are evident in these images? There is compression of the intervertebral space between nine vertebral bodies adjacent to the swim bladder. Moderate vertical displacement ('step lesion') is visible on the lateral view in the center of the affected area.

2 What is a possible etiology for this injury? The incident in this case was not observed, but trauma was suspected, most likely a result of the fish colliding head-on with an exhibit wall or décor, following a startling event.

CASE 156

1 What diagnostic tests are indicated? A CBC, chemistry panel, radiographs, coelomic ultrasound, and coelomocentesis with fluid analysis, cytology, Gram stain, acid-fast stain, and culture are all indicated as part of the initial work-up. Other testing may include a skin scrape, gill clip, fecal, and blood culture. Your initial work-up may be limited due to field conditions. Diagnostic test results were:
- Skin scrape: NSF.
- Gill clip: NSF.
- PCV/TS: 19%, 1.8 g/dL – mild anemia and moderate hypoproteinemia.
- Electrolyte panel: NSF.
- Blind coelomocentesis: 12 mL fluid removed.
- Fluid analysis: clear, colorless, TS: 0.4 g/dL.
- Fluid cytology: very low cellularity, four large mononuclear cells and three small mononuclear cells identified, no evidence of neoplasia or infectious etiologic agents. Fluid consistent with a transudate.
- Fluid Gram stain: no bacteria identified.
- Fluid acid-fast stain: no acid-fast organisms identified.

The fish was treated with enrofloxacin (10 mg/kg ICe) followed by daily enrofloxacin baths (5 mg/L × 2 hours) and metronidazole baths (25 mg/L × 2 hours). The pond was treated with 2 ppt salt.

2 What is the prognosis? A definitive diagnosis has not yet been reached, but long-term prognosis is likely poor due to concurrent hypoproteinemia, coelomic effusion, and cutaneous edema. Additional diagnostic tests would be necessary to obtain a diagnosis and provide a more accurate prognosis.

CASE 157

1 What diagnostic tests are indicated? Recheck bloodwork and imaging studies such as radiographs and coelomic ultrasound are indicated.

Diagnostic test results:
- CBC: marked anemia (PCV = 9%), low-normal leukocyte count (18.5 × $10^3/\mu L$), relative neutropenia (23%), relative lymphopenia (63%).

- Chemistry panel: marked panhypoproteinemia (TP = 0.6 g/dL, albumin = 0.2 g/dL, globulin = 0.4 g/dL), hypocalcemia (6.9 mg/dL), hypocholesterolemia (40 mg/dL), decreased AST (260 U/L), increased CK (28,1000IU/L), hyperglycemia (146 mg/dL).

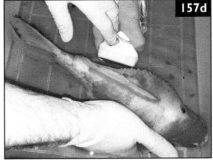

157d

- Coelomic ultrasound (**157d**): hyperechoic material present in the caudal coelomic cavity suggesting a partially mineralized mass.

- CT scan: mineralization and free coelomic fluid in the area of the gonad. A partially mineralized gonadal mass is considered most likely.

2 What treatment options will you recommend? Coelomic exploratory surgery should be recommended. Coelomic exploratory surgery was declined due to cost and likely poor prognosis. Euthanasia was also declined. Treatment with enrofloxacin and metronidazole baths was re-instituted.

3 What is the prognosis? Prognosis for survival and healing following surgery is likely poor due to the degree of anemia and hypoproteinemia present. Long-term prognosis will also be impacted by the extent of disease, which can only be determined at surgery. Furthermore, a gonadal mass does not fully explain the degree of anemia and hypoproteinemia in this animal, and addressing the mass may not resolve these problems.

4 What other diagnostic tests are indicated? Recheck bloodwork is indicated. A CBC and chemistry panel were performed. A cloacal flush was performed for a fecal float and direct evaluation due to persistent, severe hypoproteinemia identified on the bloodwork.

- CBC: progressive anemia (PCV 7%), leukocytosis (33.75 × 10³/μL) with relative neutrophilia (33%) and left shift (10% bands), relative monocytosis (2.4%), and relative lymphopenia (54%).

- Chemistry panel: marked panhypoproteinemia (TP = 0.5 g/dL, albumin = 0.2 g/dL, globulin = 0.3 g/dL), hypocalcemia (6.5 mg/dL), hypophosphatemia (2.8 mg/dL), elevated AST (1,458 U/L), increased CK (134,704 IU/L), hyperglycemia (92 mg/dL).

- Fecal float: NSF.
- Fecal direct: NSF.

5 What treatments are recommended? Systemic antibiotics are indicated due to evidence of infection. Continued antibiotic baths are indicated to topically medicate the corneal ulcer.

Answers

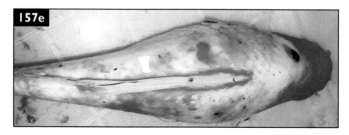

The fish was treated with ceftiofur (20 mg/kg ICe q 14 days × three treatments), enrofloxacin baths were continued, and metronidazole baths were discontinued. She showed marked improvement with this treatment regimen (**157e**). By the third ceftiofur injection, her clinical signs had completely resolved. She was eating, swimming normally, and observed spawning in the spring. While coelomic distension and 'pineconing' are conditions typically associated with a poor prognosis, the condition resolved with antibiotic therapy in this case. The suspected gonadal mass was likely an incidental finding.

CASE 158

1 What is the probable diagnosis and cause? The amount of sodium thiosulfate should measure 7 mg per 1 mg of chlorine used. In this case, not enough sodium thiosulfate was used in an effort to stretch the remnants of the last bag on the farm and the employees did not understand the consequences of their actions. This case illustrates the importance of having standards of protocol in place and ensuring that all farm employees read and understand them. About 4 weeks earlier the vats were improperly neutralized and trace amounts of bleach entered the biofilter, killing the nitrifying bacteria and resulting in an ongoing and extended 'new tank syndrome' scenario. The increased cases of columnaris disease are secondary to the ammonia toxicity affecting the fish and along with the high ammonia levels are contributing to the rise in mortality.

2 How would you manage this situation? Daily 25–50% water changes within the systems should be performed until the unionized ammonia levels fall below 0.05 mg/L. Zeolite or nitrifying bacteria can be added and the systems can also be seeded with biological filtration media from an already established system; however, it should be noted that there is the potential to introduce pathogens with this method. In this case, employees became educated on the necessity for proper dosing of sodium thiosulfate and chlorine test kits are used more routinely to ensure proper dechlorination.

CASE 159

1 Name the cells indicated by the letters and arrows. A, erythrocyte; B, thrombocyte; C, lymphocyte; D, heterophil.

CASE 160

1 How would you proceed? Begin with a thorough physical examination. The entire bloodstock cohort revealed no outward signs of disease.

2 What diagnostic imaging may help diagnose urinary bladder stones? The decision was made to screen all nine of the broodstock for stones with radiographs and ultrasonography. Two of the nine fish (22%) were diagnosed with urinary bladder stones (**160b,** right lateral radiograph of southern flounder revealing radiopaque mineral opacity urinary bladder calculi; note the metal opacity of an implanted microchip in the dorsal musculature and the round soft tissue opacity artifact in the caudal dorsal musculature due to variation in thickness of the plastic bin in which the fish is positioned; **160c,** ultrasound image of urinary calculi [arrow] within the urinary bladder [B] as seen during screening with a 6.5 MHz probe using the enclosure water as contact media (BW indicates body wall). These two fish were sacrificed following phlebotomy and additional diagnostics (**160d,** necropsy photo revealing tan urinary calculi [arrows] within the incised and reflected urinary bladder [B]; the GI tract has been removed though the kidneys [K] and heart [H] remain *in situ*). One additional fish was suspected to have urinary bladder grit, but not confirmed to have any appreciable stones. The CBC and blood chemistry values were in line with accepted reference ranges for a wide range of marine species.

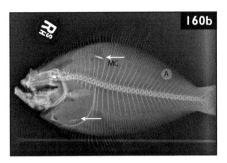

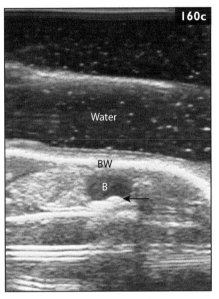

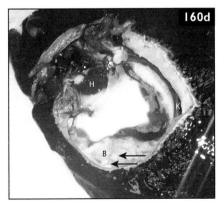

CASE 161

1 What possible etiologies may be playing an underlying role in this disease presentation? The lack of evidence of gross pathology in either fish examined suggests that although urinary bladder stone formation can occur in southern flounder, in the absence of other identified etiologies, the condition could be a response in a subset of fish to low salinity conditions. However, the pathogenesis of the stone formation found in these cases is not clear. Cation imbalance due to low salinity acclimation of fish species evolved to live in high salinity as adults, genetic predisposition of this particular subset of individuals, or underlying renal or gill dysfunction may be the underlying etiology. All stones were evaluated as calcium based, either brushite or calcium phosphate carbonate.

CASE 162

1 Review appropriate injection sites applicable to most fish. The most commonly used sites are intramuscular (IM), intracoelomic (ICe), and intravenous (IV). The image (**162a**) shows two IM options (arrows), just behind the dorsal fin (midline) and along the epaxial musculature. The former site is preferred as there is less risk of scale injury or removal. This figure also illustrates one ICe approach and the anesthetized koi has produced a fecal sample. Both the ICe approach at the base

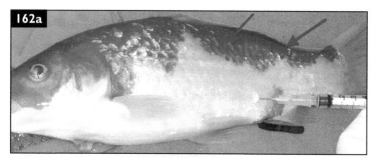

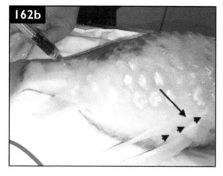

of the pelvic fin (this area is frequently devoid of scales) and IV access (a blood draw in this case) are shown here (**162b**, arrow shows location and arrowheads the angle of injection).

2 Discuss why the subcutaneous route is not commonly used. Most fish have very little subcutaneous space, making such a procedure anatomically and technically challenging.

CASE 163

1 What disease are these findings highly suggestive of? This microscopic presentation is highly suggestive of columnaris disease caused by *Flavobacterium columnare*. *F. columnare* is pathogenic at temperatures greater than ~15°C (59°F) causing erythema, ulceration, and mortality with increasing morbidity and mortality as water temperature and hardness increase.

2 What treatment protocol would you suggest and what recommendations would you make prior to restocking the system? Columnaris is primarily an epithelial disease, allowing for successful treatment with antiseptic baths if the disease is diagnosed early. Prolonged immersion in potassium permanganate or copper sulfate has been used successfully. Systemic antibiotics such as oxytetracycline are warranted in advanced cases that include dermal ulcerations. Unfortunately, in this case, all but three fish died. Recommendations to cycle the system with distilled water and potassium permanganate was made prior to new life support water and reintroduction of fish. A potassium permanganate or copper sulfate prolonged immersion is recommended during quarantine for many new fish. A preintroduction examination can be carried out on a representative sample of the newly quarantined fish to screen for *F. columnare*.

CASE 164

1 What disease is at the top of your differential list? Koi (or carp) pox disease is actually caused by a herpesvirus (*Cyprinid herpesvirus*-1). This rarely fatal disease is frequently self-limiting and usually resolves when pond temperatures increase during warmer months.

2 What conditions should also be considered? Rule-outs include neoplasia (sarcoma, squamous cell carcinoma), epitheliocystis, and lymphocystis.

3 How can you confirm the diagnosis? Diagnosis is usually based on clinical presentation, histopathology, and PCR analysis.

4 How will you manage the problem? This disease is normally cosmetic in nature, although severe lesions can result in scarring. When water temperatures rise above 25°C (77°F) the lesions usually resolve but positive fish may remain carriers. Inform the client that lesions may recur in the fall and winter but there probably is not much he can do except wait for warm water, heat the pond, or remove affected fish.

CASE 165

1 What is a sponge filter and how does it function? Sponge filters combine mechanical and biological filtration in an efficient, inexpensive, and effective manner. They are generally connected to an air pump and the forced air pulls

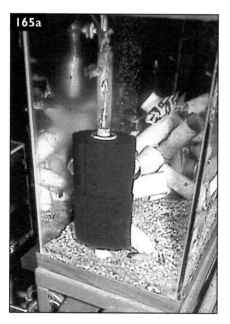

water through the high surface area inorganic sponge, which is anchored by a weight (**165a**). The sponge matrix collects debris and serves as an ideal substrate for nitrifying bacteria and other microorganisms involved in the nitrification process.

2 How can sponge filters be employed to increase biosecurity? Sponge filters are ideal for providing instant and safe biological filtration for newly acquired fish and invertebrates. These filters can be maintained in a clean system, without animals or plants, and 'fed' ammonium chloride to establish and maintain the biological filter (**165b**). When needed they can quickly and easily be employed to meet the biological demand of the system.

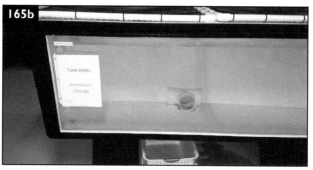

CASE 166

1 What would be on your differential list for the cause of death? Hypoxia, supersaturation disease, hyperthermia, hypothermia.

2 How could you make the diagnosis? Perform tests on the water and carry out necropsies. In this case, the cause of death was most certainly hypoxia. The DO levels were measured at 3.0 ppm and all other water parameters were within expected limits. The hypoxia resulted from the water back up and loss of the vigorous aeration that had been present prior to the carbon bag addition. The water in the unaffected pool had a DO level of 8.0 ppm.

3 **How could the DOC accumulation be managed better and safer?** Other than appearance, DOC is not a big problem for the short term. It can be managed in several ways:
- Water changes can dilute the DOC and keep levels low.
- Protein skimming (foam fractionation) can catch and remove the DOC with the protein slime that produces the foam.
- Activated carbon can be added appropriately to adsorb the DOC.

CASE 167
1 **What is UV filtration and how does it work?** UV filtration utilizes UV light produced by special bulbs that emit light in the 254 nm region of the spectrum. This light is highly toxic to most microorganisms, including viruses, bacteria, algae, fungi, yeasts, and many protozoans and their life stages. The bulbs require about the same amount of energy as a standard incandescent light bulb and are generally housed in a quartz cylinder. Water passing around the cylinder is exposed to the UV light and organisms that are exposed to the light die because of DNA alteration. A UV filter and other important life support components of a recirculating system are shown (**167**).

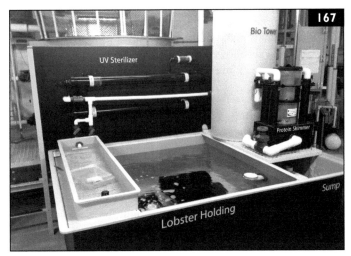

2 **What are some disadvantages and limitations of this technology?** The disadvantages of UV filtration include expense, maintenance and replacement of bulbs, and the false sense of security this technology may provide. Bulb strength and water flow rates are factors that influence efficacy. If the bulbs are older than 6 months and/or the flows are too high, then incomplete disinfection may occur.

Answers

CASE 168

1 Calculate the level of malathion present in the pond. Calculations:

50% malathion = 50 g malathion/100 mL = 500 mg malathion/mL

1 oz = 30 mL

30 mL*(500 mg/mL) = 15,000 mg malathion per 1oz administered to the pond.

15,000 mg + 22,500 mg + 45,000 mg = 82,500 mg malathion total administered to the pond.

1 US gal = 3.78 L

5,000 US gallons = 18,927 L

82,500 mg malathion/18,900 L = 4.3 mg malathion/L

Deaths have been reported at malathion levels of 0.1–30 mg/L

2 What testing could be pursued to confirm your diagnosis? Organophosphate levels can be determined in water samples and tissues (blood, liver, brain). Depressed cholinesterase levels can be demonstrated in blood and brain tissues; however, reference ranges are not available in koi.

No gross lesions were noted at necropsy. Whole blood, liver, and brain samples were saved from all the fish; however, the owners approved testing of water samples only. Unfortunately, approval for this test was delayed. Water testing was suspicious for organophosphate breakdown products, but this could not be confirmed due to degradation of the sample. Malathion is relatively labile in the environment, so degradation of the drug does not rule out toxicity. The loss of the flow-through system likely allowed malathion to concentrate to lethal levels in this case. The skin ulcers were an unrelated problem.

CASE 169

1 What potential outcomes could result from this ingestion? (1) The fish may regurgitate the foreign object independently without harm. (2) The object may pass through the stomach and into the intestines, becoming a life-threatening obstruction. (3) The object may remain in the stomach long term, resulting in discomfort and/or damage to the gastric mucosa.

2 What diagnostics and/or interventions might be necessary to ensure the well-being of this fish? Imaging in the form of radiographs or ultrasound may inform caretakers of the location of the foreign object and/or evidence of intestinal obstruction. If available, endoscopic equipment would allow for direct visualization of the stomach and foreign object. In this case, the fish did not regurgitate the plastic bottle during 2 weeks of close observation, but otherwise fed normally and appeared healthy. It was anesthetized for handling, and ultrasound of the stomach revealed distinct shadowing consistent with the

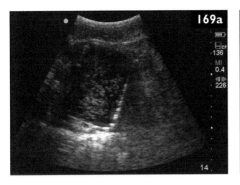

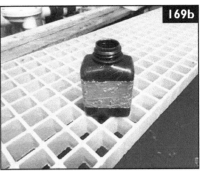

missing bottle (**169a**). The object was manually removed from the stomach through the oral cavity without incident (**169b**).

CASE 170

1 What is the most likely diagnosis? *Chilodonella* sp. These freshwater ciliates are readily identified by their shape and motion.

2 Why have the over the counter (OTC) treatments been unrewarding? As a protozoan this organism is unlikely to be susceptible to antibiotics. While Melafix® is a popular general treatment option among hobbyists, there is no evidence it acts as a parasiticide.

3 How would you manage this case? Immersion parasiticides such as formalin are usually quite effective and safe when used at the appropriate concentration. An immersion concentration of 25 ppm for 12–24 hours followed by a 30–50% water change and good supportive care will usually result in clearance of the parasites. Post-treatment biopsies can verify the treatment efficacy. Silver hatchets are sensitive fish and despite best efforts this clinical presentation will likely see few survivors. Prevention with careful screening, good biosecurity, and life support system hygiene is the best management strategy.

CASE 171

1 What type of organism is this and briefly review its natural history? This is a monogenean, a type of parasitic flatworm. Sometimes monogeneans are inaccurately referred to as monogenetic trematodes or flukes (they are neither). These parasites possess a multiple hooked attachment organ called an opisthaptor that disrupts the integrity of the host's skin and mucous membranes. Monogeneans can complete their entire life cycle on a single host and in some species the cycle may be as short as 60 hours if environmental conditions are optimal. Most species are egg layers but one family is predominantly live bearing. Crowding and other stress factors predispose ornamental fish to monogenean problems.

2 Can you identify it by taxonomic family, and if so, how? Based on the morphology this monogenean is a member of the Gyrodactylidae. This family of monogeneans contains mostly livebearers (the other three major families are egg layers). Distinctive anatomic features include a single pair of opisthaptor anchors, 16 marginal hooks, and the lack of eye spots.

3 Would you institute therapy, and if so, what regimen would you choose? In low numbers monogeneans pose little threat to the fish. In fact, it is likely that in the wild they help to remove bits of sloughing tissue and cells from the host. Unfortunately, when the host is stressed or compromised, the monogeneans can multiply quickly, overwhelming the host defenses and causing a disease state. Treating based on the presence of one or two monogeneans in a low-power field is a judgment call based on experience and the owner's input. When present in moderate to high numbers (**171b**) treatment is necessary. Praziquantel immersion therapy is the recommended

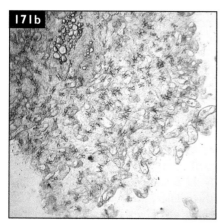

course of therapy for ornamental fish (this drug is not approved for use in food fish). Dosing regimens vary, and a formulary or colleague should be consulted where necessary, but concentrations of 2–5 mg/L for 7–15 days is generally effective. Higher doses are used for shorter time periods. Monogeneans are usually resistant to low doses of formaldehyde and even some organophosphates. Freshwater monogeneans can be killed with a 3–5 minute saltwater bath (30–35 ppt) but this does not address the eggs and/ or developmental stages that may be in the environment. Potassium permanganate and hydrogen peroxide can also be effective.

CASE 172

1 In 172a what is the structure and what are the organisms seen within and around it? Swim bladder.

2 What are your diagnosis and recommendation? The fish were diagnosed with a severe pneumocystitis. The swimbladder contains numerous roundworm eggs (presumptive capillarid) with a few juveniles noted (**172a, b**). Note the bipolar plugs in the ova (**172b**). No adult worms were observed on histopathology, so the method of infestation is in question. Based on the location of the infestation and the overwhelming presence of eggs, use of anthelmintics (i.e. levamisole or fenbendazole) is likely to be unrewarding. Depopulation and sterilization should be recommended. Attempts to determine nematode species and life cycle will assist in prevention. Broodstock and current ponds should be sampled as well.

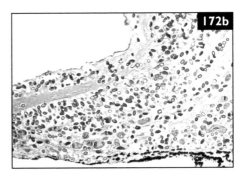

The infestation is severe enough that it most likely served as a chronic stressor, resulting in immunosuppression that facilitated reinfections of *F. columnare*.

CASE 173

1 What are these organisms? These are copepod parasites belonging to the genus *Salmonicola*. All three are mature females with paired egg sacs. These parasites can be found on the gills, skin, or fins. The copepod feeds on fluids and tissues and can be problematic for the fish, especially when they affect the gills.

2 How would you manage this issue? *Salmonicola*, like other crustacean fish parasites, undergo a direct life cycle. The eggs hatch into infective larvae that must find a fish host within several days or they die. In this case, management would involve manually removing the visible parasites and treating the quarantine system with a chitin inhibitor such as diflubenzuron or lufenuron. The aquarist should be commended for adhering to an effective quarantine protocol and preventing this parasite from entering the public display system.

CASE 174

1 What koi pond predator(s) are known to cause this sort of damage? Potential predators of koi include raccoons, canids, birds of prey, wading birds, alligators, and otters. Otters are particularly voracious predators and frequently chew the heads, tails, and fins of prey before catching another and repeating the process and leaving mutilated uneaten fish behind.

2 The client wants to know if this koi can be saved and asks you whether or not it should it be euthanized? Euthanasia was discussed with the client. While this patient was severely injured, it was alert and active, so it was hospitalized and treatment was attempted.

3 How would you treat and rehabilitate this fish? It was housed in a 380 L (100 US gal) stock tank maintained with a salt level of 0.1% at 21°C (70°F).

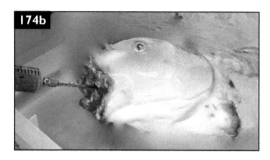

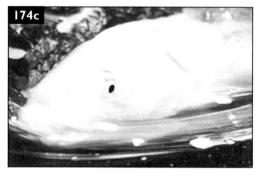

It was treated with enrofloxacin 10 mg/kg ICe q 48 hours for two doses, and then PO q 48 hours for five additional doses (14 days total). The koi was tube-fed a commercial aquatic gel diet, 3 cc/kg q 24–48 hours (174b). Even after losing its lips, the patient appeared able to 'inhale' food. After 30 days in the hospital the patient was placed back into the pond with the other koi. Eventually the fish was observed to feed on its own with the aid of a floating ring containing floating koi pellets. Seven years later the fish has a good quality of life, is able to feed on its own, and swims in an eel-like manner (174c).

CASE 175

1 **What is the most likely diagnosis?** *Brooklynella* sp. These marine ciliates are readily identified by their shape and motion.

2 **Why have the OTC treatments been unrewarding?** As a protozoan, this organism is unlikely to be susceptible to antibiotics.

3 **How would you manage this case?** Immersion parasiticides, such as formalin, are usually quite effective and safe when used at the appropriate concentration. In this case, an immersion concentration of 25 ppm for 12–24 hours followed by a 30–50% water change and good supportive care will usually result in clearance of the parasites. Post-treatment biopsies can verify the treatment efficacy.

CASE 176

1 **Describe the taxonomy of the horseshoe crab.** Horseshoe crabs belong to the phylum Arthropoda, subphylum Chelicerata, along with the arachnids. They are not crustaceans and are not related to true crabs. There are four extant species of horseshoe crab, all within the family Limulidae.

2 **What type of organism is shown on the images?** These are colonial hydroid coelenterates.

3 What treatments might help reduce or eliminate this infection? Freshwater dips are likely to be the most effective treatment and are well tolerated by these euryhaline animals. With any freshwater dip, it is essential to match pH and temperature. Mechanical débridement by gently scraping the lesions and improving environmental hygiene may help reduce loads.

CASE 177

1 What materials will you need? Standard syringes and needles should work fine. For an animal this size an insulin syringe would be ideal.

2 Where will you advise the researcher to place the syringe and needle? The peristomial membrane is soft, pliable, and easily accessible in this and related species of sea urchins (**177b**).

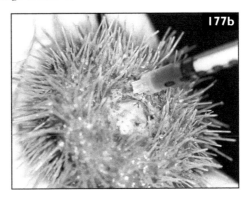

3 Can you estimate how much hemolymph you can take at each sampling time point? The standard '1% rule' can apply to sea urchins, meaning, one should be able to safely collect a total of 1.0 ml from these animals. Since the researcher wants to collect monthly samples, you should advise her to only collect the amount needed for her work, reducing the chance of complications with repeated collections.

CASE 178

1 What infectious disease is at the top of your differential list? Koi herpesvirus (KHV). This deadly disease is caused by Cyprinid herpesvirus-3. It affects carp and koi and there is evidence that other cyprinids such as goldfish can be non-clinical carriers. Clinical signs may include branchitis, branchial hemorrhage, branchial necrosis, lethargy, enophthalmia, and high mortality.

2 How would you confirm your suspicions? Several laboratories perform the necessary tests for diagnosis. Viral isolation (from spleen and/or caudal kidney; usually lethal) on a susceptible cell line such as Koi Fin (KF) is the gold standard. Non-lethal direct PCR can be performed on blood, gill tissue biopsies, and even feces. Non-lethal indirect enzyme-linked immunosorbent assay and virus neutralization can be applied to blood. A positive indirect result only indicates a fish has produced antibodies to the virus and may not be or ever have been infected.

Answers

3 **What advice would you have for your client with regard to repopulating the pond?** After an outbreak of KHV the infected stocks should be depopulated and the environment disinfected. The virus can survive in the environment for about 3 days but can be inactivated by a number of methods including sodium hypochlorite (200 ppm for 1 hour), quaternary ammonium (500 ppm for 1 hour), pH extremes of <4.0 or >10.00, and heating at 60°C (140°F) for 15 minutes. Fish obtained for repopulation should be from a confirmed KHV-free facility and quarantined for at least 30 days.

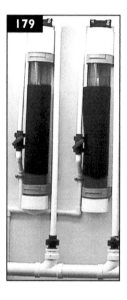

CASE 179

1 **What is a fluidized sand filter and how does it function?** Collectively, sand grains have a lot of surface area, and when vigorously aerated and agitated, provide the ideal medium for biological filtration. Typically, a clear cylinder partially filled with sand is used and a pump forces water up into the column (**179**).

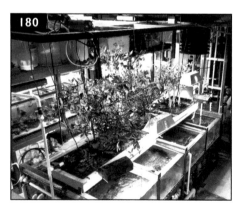

CASE 180

1 **What is a mangrove filter, how does it work, and what are the advantages and disadvantages?** A mangrove filter is a type of natural filter occasionally employed to help remove nitrates from reef systems. The plants must be carefully nurtured, but when everything is in balance, mangroves can be a beautiful behind the scenes or even visible addition to a life support system (**180**). The roots fix nitrogen,

thus keeping nitrate levels manageable. The disadvantages are that the plants may not be easy to obtain legally and they require an appropriate UV spectrum.

CASE 181

1 What are these strutures? This is a monogenean ova. The anchor-like structure would be important to a monogenean taxonomist for a more specific identification.

2 What are the clinical implications? There are likely viable and mature monogeneans in the system. This means that even if fish are not showing signs, they should be examined and a management decision made.

3 How would you manage this situation? In most cases such a finding warrants immersion therapy with praziquantel or another chemotherapeutic. With the aquarists help you examine some fish in the system and find more ova and a monogenean on a skin scraping (**181b**). You elect a 2-week course of 3 mg/L praziquantel with check up biopsies at 7 and 14 days.

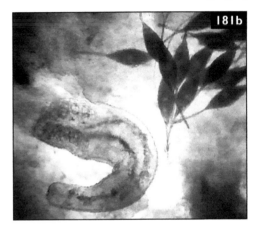

CASE 182

1 What is at the top of your differential list and what diagnostic tests would you like to perform? The clinical signs described are likely due to sea star wasting disease (SSWD). A variety of diagnostics can be performed to aid in the diagnosis of this condition; however, histopathology is definitive. Figure **182d** shows a clinically normal ochre sea star (*Pisaster ochraceus*) (left, dark purple) next to a stage 1 disease ochre sea star defined by pale appearance and distended/bloated appearance of rays and flattened central disc. The animals with the full-thickness lesions (**182a, b**) should be euthanized and

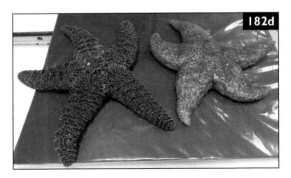

submitted for histopathology. The purple spots on the leather stars (**182c**) are likely due to pedicellariae from sea stars in the family Asteriidae. Pedicellariae from ochre stars for example are known to 'attack' stars of other species during times of stress such as capture or disease.

2 What steps should you take to reduce morbidity and mortality in the echinoderms? Isolating the asterids from other echinoderms can be helpful in reducing the morbidity and mortality of SSWD. There is no one single proven effective treatment for SSWD but options include cooling the water/increasing the DO, antibiotic baths with trimethoprim sulfa or enrofloxacin, or intracoelomic injections of enrofloxacin. The affected animals should be isolated and treated in quarantine from other areas that house echinoderms. The pedicellariae should be physically removed from the outer surface of the leather stars and the leather stars placed away from other species until any clinical abnormalities are resolved.

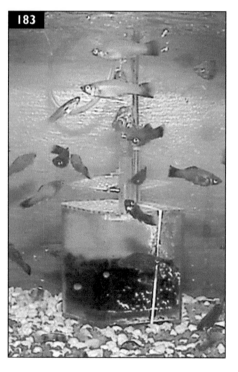

183

CASE 183

1 What is activated carbon and how does is work? Activated carbon is a specially treated form of charcoal that adsorbs and effectively removes organic contaminants and other compounds from water (and air). This technology is many decades old and still has application for life support in aquatic systems. Generally, the carbon is placed within a filter, either loose or in a mesh bag, where it is constantly submerged in still or flowing water. The carbon is in a simple box filter powered by an air line (**183**).

2 Are there any disadvantages of using activated carbon? It is believed that once activated carbon becomes saturated it can then discharge waste materials back into the water column. In addition, lignite activated carbon has been linked to gross head and lateral line erosion lesions in ocean surgeonfish (*Acanthurus bahianus*). The same study found that pelleted carbon was linked to microscopic lesions only.

CASE 184

1 What is the most likely diagnosis? Infection with *Tetrahymana corlissi*, commonly called 'guppy killer disease.' *Tetrahymena* is a ciliated protozoan that can be free-living or parasitic. The problem is common in crowded conditions and in water containing excessive organic debris.

2 Why have the OTC treatments been unrewarding? The organism is unaffected by parasiticides because of its ability to burrow deeply into the skin of the host, protecting these parasites from chemotherapeutics.

3 How would you manage this case? The best method of control is prevention through sound husbandry practices. This includes good water quality, nutrition, and environmental hygiene.

CASE 185

1 What is zeolite and how does is work? Zeolite, or more accurately zeolites, are porous volcanically produced rocks that are highly absorbent. The word comes from the Greek word 'zeo,' which means to boil, and lite, which means stone. When zeolite that is holding water is heated it releases steam, hence the name. Zeolites occur naturally but are also produced synthetically for commercial purposes. Zeolites readily accommodate the cations Ca^{2+}, K^+, Mg^{2+}, and Na^+; these are easily exchanged for other molecules such as ammonia, making zeolite an excellent adsorbing material in an aquatic life support system. One g of zeolite can remove about 1.5 g of ammonia. Zeolite can be 'recharged' by soaking it overnight in a 5% salt solution and rinsing thoroughly with fresh water. Zeolite also provides a good surface area for nitrifying bacteria but should not be used in a new system as it can make ammonia and nitrite unavailable for the developing biological filter. A bag of zeolite on top of some activated carbon and a sponge in an out-of-tank power filter is shown (**185**).

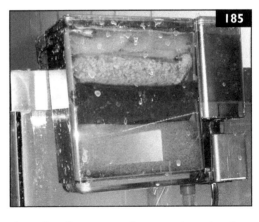

2 When would the use of zeolite be recommended? Zeolite is used to remove toxins and other compounds from an aquatic system. Excess ammonia, nitrite, nitrate, and certain chemicals are adsorbed and sequestered by zeolite.

Answers

CASE 186
1 How would you recommend treating discharge water from a 1,000 L (264 US gal) hospital tank where fish were treated with an immersion protocol of praziquantel? The most effective and economical method for removing medications from effluent is activated carbon. Zeolite or other adsorbent materials may also be employed. The exact amount of carbon required will depend on the concentration of drug in the water and exposure time to the carbon. Before instituting such a protocol one should consult a proper reference or colleague familiar with the process. Once the process is complete the used carbon can be discharged with municipal waste in most cases.

2 Would this protocol be acceptable for other types of medications? Yes, in general, but if there are questions, the recommendation is to consult local authorities familiar with the specific laws and guidelines. In the USA the Environmental Protection Agency is a good starting point.

CASE 187
1 What are these diseases? Koi herpesvirus (KHV) and spring viremia of carp (SVC).

2 Discuss their similarities and differences. Both affect carp and goldfish, are highly infectious, and are transmitted horizontally. KHV disease is caused by a herpesvirus (Cyprinid herpesvirus-3) and SVC is caused by a rhabdovirus (*Rhabdovirus carpio*).

3 Where can one find updates and further information about notifiable diseases? The OIE web site is *oie.int*. Here one can find the most current information on listed (notifiable) diseases for all taxa including fish. The 2016 listed fish diseases are given below:

- Epizootic hematopoietic necrosis.
- Infection with *Aphanomyces invadans* (epizootic ulcerative syndrome).
- Infection with *Gyrodactylus salaris*.
- Infection with HPR-deleted or HPR0 infectious salmon anemia virus.
- Infection with salmonid alphavirus.
- Infectious hematopoietic necrosis.
- Koi herpesvirus disease.
- Red sea bream iridoviral disease.
- Spring viremia of carp.
- Viral hemorrhagic septicemia.

CASE 188
1 What are your differentials? Electrocution (lightning, pump or light fixture short circuit), spinal trauma, buoyancy problem, toxin, and water quality issue. Acute onset following an electrical storm suggests lightning strike in this case.

2 How would you diagnose this case? Water quality testing (especially ammonia); radiographs. Radiographs of the patient (**188b**) indicated a spinal fracture located midway between the pectoral and anal fins.

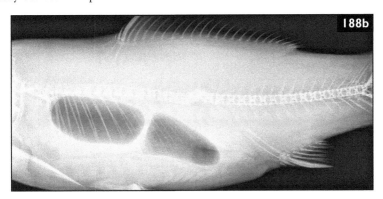

3 What are your recommendations to this client? Depending on the location (i.e. how cranial or caudal) and severity of a spinal lesion, as well as the ability of the patient to compensate, recommendations may range from conservative therapy to euthanasia. If the affected fish spends most or all of its time on the bottom, then a sinking food pellet should be recommended; otherwise, affected fish may continue to do well with floating pellets. In this case, the client elected euthanasia.

CASE 189

1 Comment on the difference between the two brains in 189. The brain on the left appears more or less normal but there is obvious hemorrhage at the base of the brain and involving the spinal cord of the brain on the right.
2 Identify the anatomic features of the brain that are numbered. 1, cerebrum (telencephalon); 2, optic lobe; 3, cerebellum; 4, medulla (myelencephalon); 5, spinal cord.
3 What anterior lobe of the brain is not clearly evident or labeled? The olfactory lobe and nerves are not clear but are located just rostral to the cerebrum (1).

CASE 190

1 What is a sand filter and how does it function? Sand filters are electrically powered units that are commonly employed to clean swimming pool water (**190**, red arrows). They are usually stout, rounded fiberglass tanks that can stand about 1 meter high and half a meter in diameter. The filter contains a large amount of

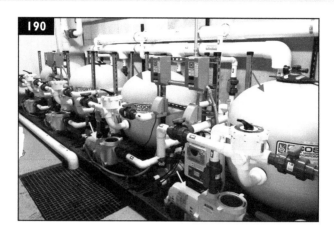

sand through which pressurized water is pumped (pumps, yellow arrows). The water flow can be reversed by the changing of a large switch to 'back wash' the sand and essentially clean the filter. This 'back wash' is sent to drain, usually as waste water. Sand filters combine mechanical and biological filtration. In order to function properly they should be back washed at least once a week depending on the organic load.

CASE 191

1 What are these 'grubs'? These organisms are most likely encysted metacercaria belonging to the genus *Clinostomum*. This genus of digenean trematode, as well as others, is common in fish reared in conditions where both snails and birds are present. The fish serves as the second intermediate host after the invertebrate (usually a gastropod) and before the definitive host, most commonly a piscivorous bird.

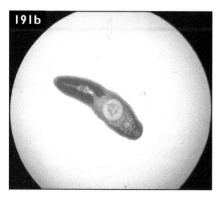

2 How can you confirm the diagnosis? Diagnosis is confirmed by excising some grubs with a clean scalpel blade or other sharp instrument and examining them with either a magnifying glass or dissecting microscope (**191b** [approximately 10× magnification]).

3 What is the risk to the fish? In general these parasites are not harmful to the fish and are more of an aesthetic problem.

4 How would you manage the problem? While individual metacercariae can be removed surgically, at the population level the problem can only be alleviated by eliminating either the avian or gastropod component of the life cycle. Covering ponds is one approach to the problem.

CASE 192

1 What is the most likely diagnosis? Infection with *Uronema* sp., a ciliated protozoan that can be free-living or parasitic. The problem is common in crowded conditions and in water containing excessive organic debris.

2 Why have the OTC treatments been unrewarding? The organism is generally unaffected by parasiticides when it is causing lesions because of its ability to burrow deeply into the skin of the host, protecting these parasites from chemotherapeutics.

3 How would you manage this case? The best method of control is prevention through sound husbandry practices. This includes good water quality, nutrition, and environmental hygiene. These practices, combined with an appropriate parasiticide such as formalin, are recommended in this case.

CASE 193

1 What is ozone filtration and how does it work? Ozone (O_3) is a gas that can be produced by an ozone generator (**193**). The gas is not stable at room temperature and cannot be held in a cylinder or other storage vessel. Ozone is usually mixed in a chamber with water from the aquatic system. Ozone is a strong oxidizing agent and this is how it kills microorganisms. A number of studies have quantified the amounts of ozone needed to kill certain types of pathogens and other organisms. When working with an ozone generator it is important to be familiar with the unit's specifications and the system requirements. A number of factors including oxidative redox potential, turbidity, biological load, and goals of ozone use come into play.

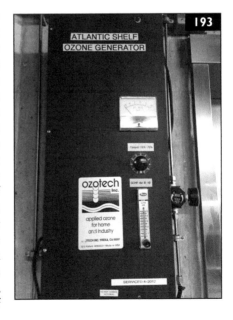

2 What are some disadvantages and limitations of this technology? The disadvantages include cost of the unit, electricity (although this is minimal), maintenance, and perhaps most importantly, risk to animals and people. Ozone is toxic to all life forms at high enough concentrations and an inappropriate applied ozone dose, ozone leak, or unit malfunction can result in unintended harmful consequences.

CASE 194

1 How would you manage this case? First isolate the affected sea star and perform tissue biopsies looking for pathogens via wet mounts and stained cytology. In this case, only bacteria were observed and the animal was placed in a 20 L

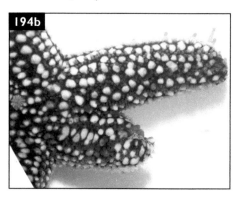

(5.2 US gal) plastic container and treated with a continuous bath of oxytetracycline (200 mg/mL stock) maintained at a concentration of 12.9 mg/L tank water for 10 days. The concentration was maintained by adding 1.2 ml stock oxytetracycline to 20 L (5.2 US gal) new tank water used in daily 75–100% water changes over the 10-day treatment interval. The lesions resolved quickly and the sea star made a full recovery (**194b**, taken 4 days after treatment began).

2 What changes would you recommend in the future during new animal accession? In the future new accessions should be separated and quarantined by species if at all possible. While there is no guarantee this would have protected the sea stars, it is possible there was disease transmission or even interspecies aggression between the echinoderms and the hermit crabs.

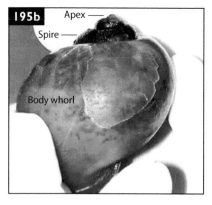

CASE 195

1 Describe gastropod shell anatomy. The shell of a typical gastropod contains the apex, spire (made up of whorls), and the body whorl, which contains the aperture (**195b**). The oldest whorls are those closest to the apex and the head and foot of the snail protrude from the aperture. The gastropod shell is composed of the outer periostracum, made of conchin, a horny protein, and the internal shell layers composed of calcium carbonate and organic material.

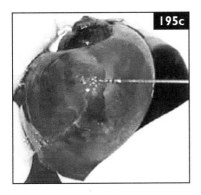

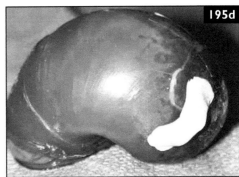

2 How would you manage this problem? The fractured shell and underlying tissues were flushed copiously with sterile saline (**195c**). An abrasive Dremel drill bit was used to roughen the surfaces on either side of the fracture. Surgical epoxy was used to construct a small bridge that was attached to the shell surface with digital pressure (**195d**). A small piece of Tegaderm™ was secured to the shell over the area of the depression fracture. The snail was

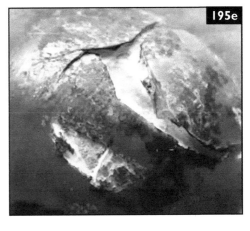

kept out of water for approximately 1 hour to allow for adhesive curing. Three months later the compromised shell sites were stable and the epoxy and Tegaderm were removed (**195e**). Despite the stability of the shell, defects persisted due to the fact that mollusks lay down shell at the free edges of the mantle. The stability of the shell is most likely due to soft tissue healing beneath the whorl.

CASE 196

1 Discuss the process of making seawater (from a commercial product). For several decades it has been easy to purchase prepared sea salts that can be dissolved in clean fresh water to form artificial seawater (**196a**). These products come with clear directions and many liters of the desired salinity can be produced in a short period of time (**196b**).

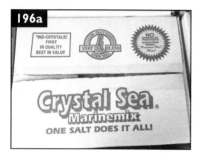

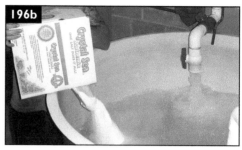

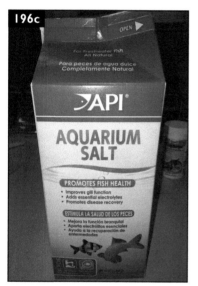

2 **What are the advantages and disadvantages compared with natural seawater?** The obvious advantage of this process is that seawater can be available virtually anywhere in the world. The product is essentially pathogen free and without contaminants. The obvious disadvantage is cost; making large volumes of seawater is expensive. Another disadvantage is the lack of microorganisms in natural seawater. These organisms contribute to the overall balance of the system and can enhance biological filtration, especially in a newly established system. It should be added that these salts can be used at much lower concentrations with therapeutic and support benefit to freshwater fish. Some companies even market salts for this purpose (**196c**).

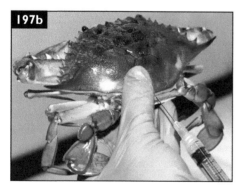

CASE 197

1 **What is this agent?** Alfaxalone.

2 **What route and dose would you use for sedation and anesthesia respectively?** Alfaxalone can be administered into the heart or pericardial sinus via the arthrodial membrane at a dose of 15 or 100 mg/kg for sedation or deep anesthesia, respectively (**197b**).

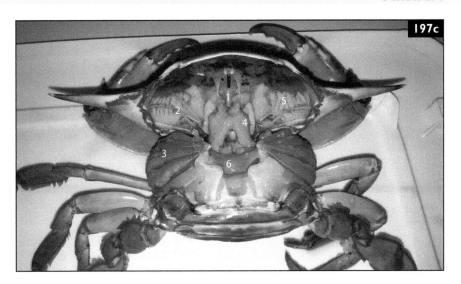

3 What organs are in close proximity to the heart and can be avoided if the syringe and needle are placed appropriately in the center of the arthrodial membrane? The hepatopancreas and gonad are the major organs surrounding the heart (**197c**: 1, stomach; 2, gill raker; 3, gill; 4, ovary; 5, digestive gland [hepatopancreas]; 6, heart).

CASE 198

1 What radiographic abnormality is detected incidental to the PIT tag position determination? Variable swim bladder shape, with soft tissue or fluid radiopacity, completely obscuring the swim bladder in one case.

2 What is the probable cause of the abnormality? *Anguillicoloides crassus*, the parasitic nematode of *Anguilla* spp. eel swim bladders.

3 What continent is the source of the responsible agent, and what impacts can it have? Asia. *Anguillicoloides crassus* infests the Japanese eel, *A. japonica*, and is invasive in Europe and North America where it now also infests European eels (*A. anguilla*) and American eels, which are more severely affected than Japanese eels. The parasite is transmitted via ingestion of intermediate and paratenic hosts (copepods, ostracods, fish). Larval stages lodge in the swim bladder wall, while adults are in the lumen where they feed on blood from vessels lining the swim bladder and can produce a brown fluid. Health effects can include anemia, negative buoyancy, reduced swimming efficiency, and death. Eels become infected at the advanced elver (glass eel) stage shortly after recruiting from the ocean into estuaries, and prevalence can range up to 80%. There is no known treatment.

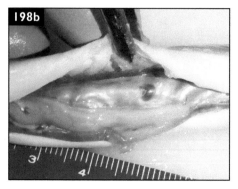

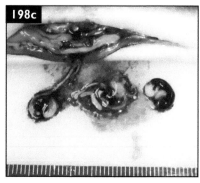

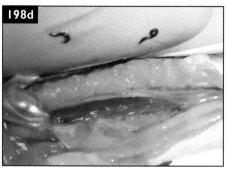

American eel swim bladder (silvery organ central in the body cavity) showing outlines of adult nematodes in the lumen bulging out against the swim bladder wall (**198b**). Image **198c** shows adult *Anguillicoloides crassus* and brown fluid from the swim bladder lumen in **198b**. Larval *Anguillicoloides crassus* from American eel swim bladder (**198d**).

CASE 199

1 Discuss the different reproductive strategies, including basic anatomy and taxonomy, of these small but popular species. Cardinal tetras are native to the Negro and Orinoco rivers, both Amazon River tributaries, and belong to the family Characidae. They are egg layers and fertilization takes place externally when the female and male gametes are simultaneously released into the water after a period of courtship. The eggs hatch in about 3 days and the fry begin feeding once the yolk supply is exhausted. In the wild it is thought the cardinal is an annual species but in captivity they can live for several years or more.

Guppies are native to northeast South America and several Caribbean islands; they belong to the family Poeciliidae. Guppies are livebearers with a modified form of internal fertilization. The males of this family possess an intromittent organ called a gonopodium, which is actually a modified anal fin for copulation and sperm transfer. The genital pore of a receptive female (they are polyandrous and thus accept multiple males) receives the gonopodium and fertilization ensues. Gestation lasts approximately 3 weeks.

CASE 200

1 What are your differential diagnoses? Electrocution (lightning, electrical fixture short circuit), spinal trauma, toxin, water quality issue.

2 What additional history would be helpful? Ask if there has been a recent electrical storm (potential close proximity lightning strike) or any electrical problems (i.e. pump or light fixture short circuit) involving the pond; any possible trauma; any chemicals used or recent changes to water treatment system. The client informs you that prior to the onset of clinical signs, an electrical problem with the pond occurred and the pump had to be replaced. Problems with the affected fish were not noticed until after this activity.

3 What diagnostic tests are needed? Water quality testing; radiographs. Radiographs (**200b**) indicated a spinal fracture located at vertebra 5, midway between the pectoral and anal fins.

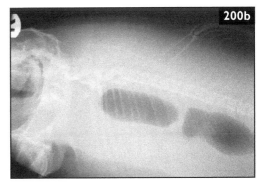

4 What are your recommendations to the client? This was most likely a case of electrocution with subsequent spinal trauma. Depending on the location (i.e. how cranial or caudal) and severity of a spinal lesion, as well as the ability of the patient to compensate, recommendations may range from conservative therapy to euthanasia. If the affected fish spends most or all of its time on the bottom, then a sinking food pellet should be recommended; otherwise, affected fish may continue to do well with floating pellets. In this case, the client elected euthanasia, which was performed by administering a prolonged overdose of tricaine methanesulfonate. (**Note:** A second step, such as pithing or cranial concussion, is recommended.) Necropsy revealed the extent of the damage (**200c**), including extensive hemorrhage ventral to the spinal fracture and surrounding the swim bladder.

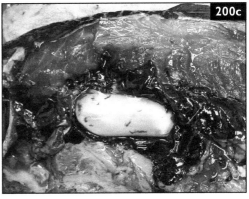

Answers

CASE 201

1 What diagnostic tests would you recommend to the owner? A basic diagnostic battery should include:

- Physical examination: no external parasites, and body condition was a body score of 3/5.
- Water quality testing: results: pH 6, ammonia 0.25, nitrite 0 ppm, nitrate 80–160 ppm.
- Gill clip: the lamellae were very pale but no evidence of parasites.
- Skin scraping: normal, no evidence of parasites.

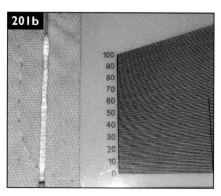

- Blood collection using heparin prepped syringe. Packed cell volume (PCV)/total solids (TS): PCV was 1.5% and TS 1.0 mg/dL (**201b**).
- Blood smear: the smear contained predominantly mature and immature erythrocytes. Leukocytes were characterized by normal numbers of small lymphocytes, mildly decreased numbers of granulocytes, and a few monocytes. Small clumps of thrombocytes were seen.

2 What rule outs would you expect for this fish? Rule outs for this fish's dyspnea could be: branchial disease, cardiovascular disease, and anemia. In this case, anemia appeared to be the cause for the dyspnea and may have been due to previous

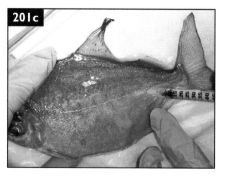

unknown trauma, chronic infection, neoplasia, a hematopoietic disorder, autoimmune disease, or sepsis. While lymph contamination was considered, the clinicians made two attempts at blood collection from the hemal arch and felt confident in their technique and that they had collected peripheral blood (**201c**). The water quality parameters are not ideal and indicate that more water changes are needed to reduce nitrates and elevate pH.

3 How would you manage this case? This fish was placed on enrofloxacin (10 mg/kg ICe q 4 days) and iron dextran (12 mg/kg IM q 7 days) in addition to regular supportive care and nutritional support. Tube feeding was considered if the anorexia persisted. Unfortunately, the fish continued to decline, was euthanized, and a presumptive hepatic carcinoma and renal granulomas were found on necropsy.

CASE 202

1 Based on the figure (202), is this animal a male or female? Actually, this is a trick question, as it is both sexes (many gastropods are hermaphroditic). The presence of an egg mass, assuming they are from this animal, means that the female tract is active but some gastropods are simultaneous hermaphrodites.

2 What is unusual about many freshwater snails compared with marine snails with regard to respiration? Many species of freshwater snails are air breathers using a structure called a pallial lung for respiration.

3 What is unusual about the hemolymph of this family compared with most other invertebrates? The oxygen carrying pigment for most members of this family is hemoglobin, in contrast to hemocyanin, the most common respiratory pigment of invertebrates.

CASE 203

1 What is foam fractionation as it pertains to water quality and life support systems? Foam fractionation is a natural process that occurs when very small air bubbles are forced into water and their collective high surface area attracts and accumulates oppositely charged organic particles such as proteins and mucopolysaccharides. Natural foam fractionation can be observed on beaches, rocky shores, and other aquatic environments where the water is high in minerals (i.e. sea water and hard fresh water). The images show normal foam fractionation in an Ecuadorian mountain stream (**203a**) and on a Galápagos beach (**203b**).

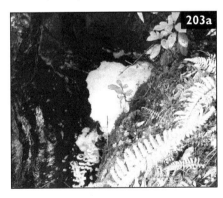

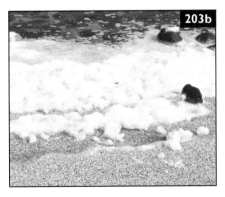

2 What is the common name for filtration units that employ this process and give an example of a system where such a unit has utility. Foam fractionation devices are normally called protein skimmers (**203c**). In these artificial systems turbulent air is injected into a downward flowing water column (Venturi effect)

Answers

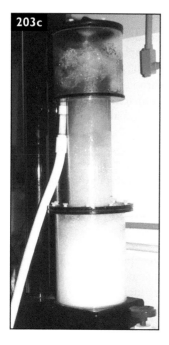

and thousands of tiny bubbles are produced that bind to organics and other appropriately charged debris. This rising column of bubbles eventually overflows into a drain. Since the waste is removed from the top of the column it is called skimming. Protein skimmers are inexpensive and efficient to operate and maintain. They are commonly employed to clean reef tanks and other marine systems.

CASE 204

1 What is your top differential based on the clinical presentation and history? Grossly, the organisms adhered to the barbels ('whiskers') of the catfish appear to be leeches (hirudineans). Another possibility would be a crustacean ectoparasite like the anchorworm.

2 Can you describe the life cycle and impact of this organism on fish? Most leeches drop from the host after taking a sufficient blood meal and then produce egg-filled cocoons that are deposited on various substrates. Leeches directly harm fish by removing blood and acting as a vector for disease.

3 How would you manage this situation? Capture the fish and give it a thorough physical examination. If leeches are confirmed, then it is possible, if not likely, that eggs or juveniles are in the system. Normally a proper quarantine would prevent this situation from occurring. In this case, there are two options. The conservative wait-and-see approach to determine if the leeches have colonized the system, and then treating accordingly, or the more aggressive treat right away approach, assuming the risk of leeches in the system is high. Leeches are notoriously hard to eradicate from a population of fish. The most effective methods include persistent trichlorfon immersion therapy complemented with manual leech removal in some cases.

CASE 205

1 What is this organism? This is an isopod parasite belonging to the family *Cymothoidae*. These parasites can be found on the gills, skin, fins, and in the case of the tongue-eating/tongue-replacing isopod, the buccal cavity. The isopod feeds on blood and can be problematic for the fish, especially when they affect the gills.
2 How would you manage this problem? Cymothoids, like other crustacean fish parasites, undergo a direct life cycle. The eggs hatch into infective larvae and then search for a host. In this case, management would involve manually removing the visible parasites and treating the quarantine system with a chitin inhibitor such as diflubenzuron or lufenuron. The aquarist should be commended for closely observing her charges and bringing this matter to your attention.

CASE 206

1 What measurements would you want to have and how would you calculate volume with these values? If you know the length, width, and average depth of the pond, the volume can be calculated by multiplying these three values (in meters or feet) to give either cubic feet or cubic liters. To determine liters multiply by 1,000 (liters/cubic meter) and to determine US gallons multiply the total by 7.48 (gal/cu ft). For example, in this case, the client's pond measures 6.1 m (20 ft) long, 3.05 m (10 ft) wide, and with an average depth of 0.91 m (3 ft). This comes to just about 17,000 L or 4,500 US gal. Many lined earthen koi ponds are irregularly shaped, thus measurements will not be exact (especially depth), and an error factor of up to 20% should be considered.
2 Can you name an alternate method that would not require any pond dimension values? One approach would be to drain the pond (at least most of the water) and refill with a steady stream from a hose. By filling a known volume container (e.g. 40–400 L; 10–100 US gal) with water from the hose and timing this process, one can then fill the pond, divide the total time by the known volume increment, and determine pond volume. For example, if it takes 5 minutes to fill a 50-US gallon drum, and it takes 450 minutes to fill the pond, the pond volume is 4,500 US gal. For very large ponds, measured in acres rather than gallons or liters, a known amount of sodium chloride can be added to the pond and then measured a day or two later to calculate volume. One acre-foot of water equals 2.71 million pounds, so 1.0 ppm salt equals 2.71 pounds. Adding this much salt to one acre-foot of pond would increase the salinity (sodium and chloride) 1.0 ppm. In order to use this method an accurate chloride test kit is required. The first step is to determine the background chloride concentration. Once that is done then a known amount of salt is broadcast into the pond (assume 50 pounds per estimated acre). After a day or two, take several chloride measurements from various areas and depths of the pond and average these values. Then use the formula: volume = (weight of salt

applied × 0.6) + 2.71 (acre-feet)/ change in chloride concentration. For example, if one added 100 pounds of salt and the measured average net (final − initial) concentration was 5.5 ppm chloride, the formula would read: 100 × 0.6 + 2.71/ 5.5 = 11.4 acre-feet.

CASE 207

1 What commonly used fish anesthetic can be used to anesthetize sea urchins and at what concentration? Tricaine methanesulfonate (MS-222) has been shown to be safe and effective for purple sea urchins, and possibly other echinoderms, at a concentration of between 0.4 and 0.8 g/L. Urchins usually dislodge their tube feet and become easy to handle after several minutes. Recovery is rapid once they are placed in clean seawater.

CASE 208

1 What is the likely source of the problem? Pressure washing solution may contain chlorine bleach (sodium hypochlorite), surfactants, detergents, acids, and/or other chemicals, all of which are potentially harmful to fish.

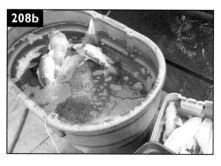

2 What steps would you take to help these fish? Immediately remove all fish from the pond and transfer them to a treatment tank containing fresh, aerated water (208b). Add salt (sodium chloride) to the treatment water at a concentration of approximately 0.12% (1.2 kg/1,000 L; 1 lb/100 US gal) to reduce osmotic stress.

3 What is the prognosis? Prognosis is poor to grave since chlorine causes acute branchial necrosis and compromises gill function. Despite aggressive supportive care all the fish in this pond were lost (208c).

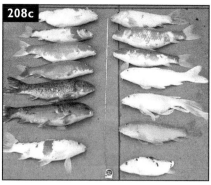

4 How would you prevent this from happening in the future? The workers attempted to prevent pressure washing solution from getting into the pond by covering the water with plastic sheeting. Unfortunately, this was not adequate, and solution either drifted into the pond or runoff flowed in. The best recommendation is to not pressure wash in close proximity to a pond containing live fish.

CASE 209

1 What is your primary differential? Koi herpesvirus (KHV) should be suspected. The virus remains latent in cold water below 17.8–20°C (64–68°F) and becomes active above 21.1°C (70°F). Affected koi may exhibit a variety of clinical signs including head down swimming, lethargy and weakness, gill necrosis, excessive slime coat, and skin lesions. KHV does not affect goldfish.

2 How would you confirm your suspicion? Diagnosis of KHV is via virus isolation (culture), DNA detection (polymerase chain reaction) and antibody detection (enzyme-linked immunosorbent assay).

3 What can you do to help the remaining fish? Increase water temperature to 30.6°C (87°F) or above; increase salinity to 0.3% or higher to combat osmotic stress; increase aeration of the water, since gills are compromised, and warm water carries less oxygen; treat with antibiotics to fight secondary bacterial infection. Surviving fish should be considered potential carriers and never moved to another pond. The same biosecurity applies to any unaffected fish, water, plants, etc. The safest approach is depopulation if KHV is confirmed and then following strict biosecurity protocols for repopulation.

4 How can the client reduce the chance of a similar event happening again? Quarantine new fish before placing them in the koi pond for at least 30 days and perform antemortem screening for KHV.

CASE 210

1 What are these organisms? These are goose barnacles (*Lepas* sp.) and are most likely commensal on the slipper lobster. Barnacles are filter feeders and may benefit from the availability of different feeding environments presented via a mobile host.

2 How would you manage this issue? While it is not known if the barnacles are causing any harm, it would be best to keep them out of the system, unless there was a good reason to do otherwise. Since both host and 'parasite' are crustaceans, chemical treatment would be risky to the lobster. A proper quarantine, manual removal, and close observation should prevent the barnacles from colonizing the exhibit.

CASE 211

1 What is this syndrome called? This captive jellyfish problem is known as eversion syndrome.

2 What is known about it? This appears to affect captive jellies in some aquaria and institutions. Young and older jellies are most vulnerable. A definitive cause has not been identified but the syndrome seems linked to husbandry in some manner. Histologically, there is muscle and mesoglea (soft tissue matrix) degeneration.

3 How would you manage the problem? Anecdotally, aquaria using natural seawater, or those keeping wild jellies, have a very low incidence, if any. You should carefully evaluate the husbandry protocols, learn as much as possible about the source of and/or propagation of the jellies, and consult with colleagues at institutions not experiencing this challenge.

CASE 212
1 Name the cells indicated by the letters and arrows. A, erythrocyte; B, heterophil (leukocyte); C, thrombocyte.

CASE 213
1 How would you anesthetize the cuttlefish for this procedure? Please include details on induction, maintenance, and recovery. Once the animal has been safely captured it should be placed in a circular induction vessel. At this point the induction concentration of an appropriate anesthetic can be administered. Ethanol at a concentration of 3% is an effective, safe, and inexpensive choice. Once the cuttlefish is unconscious it can be placed on a recirculating anesthesia system containing 1–2% ethanol. The safest option is to have a pair of tubes irrigating both sets of gills (**213**).

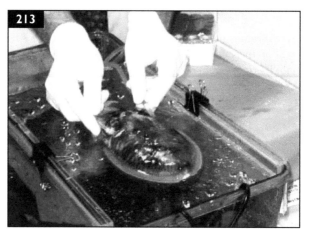

CASE 214

1 What information would you like to have before commenting? You will need to know the weight of the fish, and find out they all weigh within a gram or 2 of 40 g.

2 Based on this information how would you calculate an estimate for safe blood collection volume? One can only estimate blood volume for most fish species but it is probably between 5 and 7% of the total body weight. Thus, a 40-g fish would have between 2.0 and 2.8 ml of blood. It is generally safe to remove 10% of a fish's blood volume, meaning that for this study, 0.25 ml would be a good maximum target.

3 What anatomic site would you recommend the IACUC approved researchers use for the blood samples? The most commonly used site for blood collection in fish is the caudal vein, sometimes referred to as the hemal arch, since arterial and venous blood flow adjacent to each other. The figure (**214**) illustrates blood collection from a goldfish using the lateral approach. Some workers prefer accessing the same blood source with a ventral approach.

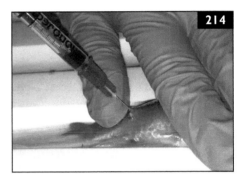

CASE 215

1 What recommendations would you have for the owner regarding safe and efficient transportation?

- Transport the fish by personal vehicle.
- Transport the fish by shipping with a next day mail service. Ideally, a next day morning arrival.
- Transport the fish as cargo on a commercial airline.

2 How would you package the fish for transport? Fish can be transported in a non-breakable container with a battery aerator and a carbon filter for ground transport as the cheapest but riskiest option (**215a**). Partial water changes are required. Air cargo or shipping by a mail service requires the fish to be packaged in a plastic bag with a water conditioner and enough water for the fish to move and at least triple their height.

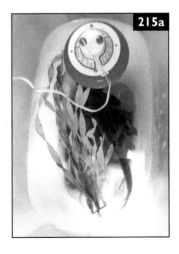

Answers

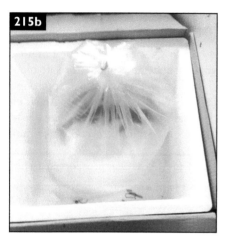

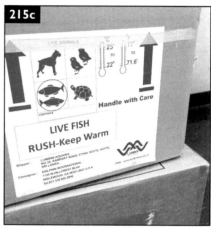

Fill the bag with oxygen and secure it with sturdy rubber bands. In most cases the bag should contain about one-third water and two-thirds oxygen. Enclose the fish bag in a second, secured plastic bag. Place the bags in a styrofoam lined box (**215b**) and properly close and label the box (**215c**). Shipping fish by mail service is the most expensive but guarantees arrival at your destination. Shipping by cargo is a middle cost option with none or one layover of 2–4 hours. There is a risk of the container being left outside if the flight is not non-stop (direct flights imply one airplane but they can stop and start again) and the fish must be picked up at airport cargo. Most airlines will provide some form of guarantee of animals arriving alive. If packed appropriately, and some fish wholesalers or advanced hobbyists can help with the packing, most boxes should be safe for 24–36 hours. It is recommended fish be held off feed for 1–2 days prior to packing.

CASE 216

1 How can this be accomplished? First you must identify the species involved and become familiar with their anatomy if you are not already. Next, a sharp drill bit large enough to accept an appropriately sized hypodermic needle should be secured to a high-speed drill, and the entry site selected (**216a**). While drilling through the shell in the direction of the pericardium, saline can be dripped onto the drill bit to reduce heat and friction. Once the shell is penetrated the sterile needle is inserted into the pericardium and hemolymph withdrawn (**216b**). The final step is to seal the breach with bone wax or another comparable water proof and non-toxic material.

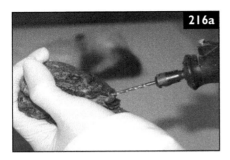
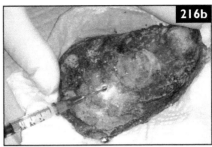

CASE 217

1 What is your primary differential for this situation? A rapid drop in pH ('pH crash') could be responsible for these losses.

2 Explain the water test results for your client. The alkalinity (carbonate level) of pond water determines its buffering capacity. Without adequate alkalinity, pond pH may suddenly drop due to heavy rainfall. Normal rain has a pH of 6.5–5.0; however, 'acid rain' can have a pH of 4.0 or lower. If this pond had only marginal carbonate levels prior to the rain, then a deluge could result in a rapid drop in pH, which severely stresses koi. Low pH also adversely affects the biofilter, causing ammonia to rise, which further stresses the fish. Without an active biofilter, nitrite is not being produced, and without regular water changes, nitrates have accumulated to higher than recommended levels.

3 What steps would you take to resolve this problem, and what special precautions should you take? Maintain salt level at 0.10–0.30% to reduce osmotic stress. One needs to remove ammonia BEFORE raising pH so as not to convert ammonium ion to toxic ammonia. Perform 50% water changes daily to remove ammonia. Place zeolite granules in the filtration system to actively absorb ammonia, and regularly 'recharge' these by soaking them in salt water to release trapped ammonia. As ammonia levels fall, slowly raise the pH in the pond with a combination of sodium bicarbonate (quick acting source of carbonate) and crushed oyster shell or crushed coral (long-acting sources of carbonate). As pH level rises to normal and ammonia levels fall, the fish should return to normal and the biofilter will begin to function.

CASE 218

1 What is a canister filter and how does it function? Canister filters are electrically powered devices that frequently combine biological, chemical, and mechanical filtration principles (**218**). They are self-contained units with a pump (usually at the top) filled with high surface area substrate for mechanical and biological filtration.

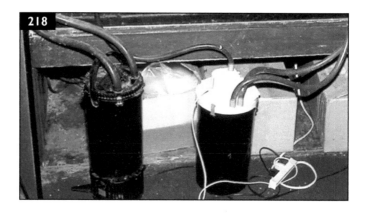

This substrate can be in the form of a cartridge that can be replaced. Some canister filters utilize inorganic chips, stones and, for chemical filtration, activated carbon or zeolite.

CASE 219

1 Obviously a number of actions are required. List them in order of priority. (1) Turn off the hose; (2) examine the animals contained in the system; and (3) test the water with priority given to salinity.

2 What precautions could be taken to prevent this from happening in the future? Establish some type of safeguard system whenever a hose is used to fill an aquarium. This could be in the form of a timed alarm, human back up person, or both. One might ask why was something as simple as a tap water hose used to supply water to an established marine exhibit. Many public aquaria have very large pipes (10–60 cm diameter) designed to move SW throughout the facilities. The SW is usually made on site and stored. In a few cases natural seawater is pumped in, filtered, and then stored. However, in many cases, these aquaria rely on a much smaller diameter pipe to move FW. The FW is usually taken directly off the domestic water main and run through a granular activated carbon filter to remove chlorine. This can become a problem when trying to rapidly adjust salinity in very large systems. Few aquaria have the capability to replace thousands of gallons of FW as quickly as they can change SW. Rather than drain water from a display system, leaving an unsightly exhibit, and stressing animals with a decreased water volume, adding clean FW from a hose can provide a gradual water change and salinity can be monitored and corrected appropriately. If the staff remain observant, there is little chance for error. There also needs to be an adequate overflow system in place so floods are avoided. There have been numerous human failures where FW has been running for hours, or in some cases overnight, into aquaria. Depending on the size of the aquarium and the flow of FW, this can be catastrophic. In this case, a check of the water chemistry showed the salinity had dropped to 18 ppt; it was 31 ppt earlier that week. The laboratory technician had tried to drop the salinity a few points the day prior, left early, and did not do a routine check before leaving. The oversight could have been fatal. Fortunately, all of the fish on the system survived, and a new operating plan was established.

3 What is a beneficial side effect of lowered salinity? A gradual, controlled reduction in salinity is a strategy to control some ectoparasites of fish. The scenario in this case would not be the way to achieve this effect; while the fish were apparently unharmed, it is possible that some parasites were also unharmed.

CASE 220

1 What intracoelomic (ICe) dosing regimen would you recommend? A dose of 10 mg/kg given ICe q 5 days should produce effective levels for most pathogens sensitive to enrofloxacin.

2 What immersion dosing regimen would be appropriate? A 6-hour immersion in 10 mg/L q 3 days should result in effective antibacterial levels of this drug.

CASE 221

1 Briefly describe a sea hare. Sea hares are marine gastropod mollusks that lack a shell. They are an important research animal for the study of neurophysiology but are also kept in aquaria as display or educational animals (**221**).

2 On your way to address the issue you stop and patiently answer a visitor's questions about one of the exhibits. Why are you not in a rush to save the hemorrhaging sea hare? Sea hares will expel a red to purple 'ink' when disturbed or agitated. While this can temporarily foul the water, the animal is not at risk and should be fine.

3 If the sea was truly 'bleeding' (losing hemolymph), what color would it be and why? The hemolymph would be a very light blue color, due to the oxygen carrying pigment hemocyanin.

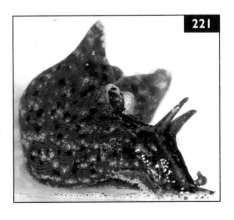

4 If you had to anesthetize a sea hare, what chemical and concentration would be appropriate? Magnesium chloride hexa-hydrate at a concentration of 50 mg/L is both safe and effective for the California sea hare. Intracoelemic magnesium sulfate has also been used in this species.

Index

Note: References are to case numbers, not page numbers.

Index

Index

Index

Index

Also available in the Self-Assessment Color Review series

Brown & Rosenthal: *Small Mammals*
Elsheikha & Patterson: *Veterinary Parasitology*
Forbes & Altman: *Avian Medicine*
Freeman: *Veterinary Cytology*
Frye: *Reptiles and Amphibians 2nd Edition*
Hartmann & Levy: *Feline Infectious Diseases*
Hartmann & Sykes: *Canine Infectious Diseases*
Keeble, Meredith & Richardson: *Rabbit Medicine and Surgery 2nd Edition*
Kirby, Rudloff & Linklater: *Small Animal Emergency and Critical Care Medicine 2nd Edition*
Lewis & Langley-Hobbs: *Small Animal Orthopedics, Rheumatology & Musculoskeletal Disorders 2nd Edition*
Mair & Divers: *Equine Internal Medicine 2nd Edition*
May & McIlwraith: *Equine Orthopaedics and Rheumatology*
Meredith & Keeble: *Wildlife Medicine and Rehabilitation*
Moriello: *Small Animal Dermatology*
Moriello & Diesel: *Small Animal Dermatology, Advanced Cases*
Obradovich: *Small animal Clinical Oncology*
Pycock: *Equine Reproduction and Stud Medicine*
Samuelson & Brooks: *Small Animal Ophthalmology*
Scott: *Cattle and Sheep Medicine 2nd Edition*
Sparkes & Caney: *Feline Medicine*
Tennant: *Small Animal Abdominal and Metabolic Disorders*
Thieman-Mankin: *Small Animal Soft Tissue Surgery 2nd Edition*
Verstraete & Tsugawa: *Veterinary Dentistry 2nd Edition*
Ware: *Small Animal Cardiopulmonary Medicine*